THE POWER OF LYMPH-CHI TREATMENT®

Unleashing the Healing Potential of the Body's Energy Systems

DR. TRACY ROSA

ISBN: 978-1-961292-16-1

ACKNOWLEDGMENT

I extend my heartfelt gratitude to Viki West, Cameron Richardson, Sandy Nunez, Jennifer Baltimore, and Gabrielle Glore for their honest review of the efficacy of this treatment. Your testimonials have greatly contributed to the credibility of this book and offered hope to others on their healing journeys.

I also want to thank all my clients for their trust and support in embracing the Lymph-Chi Treatment. Your commitment to wellness has inspired me and deepened my understanding of healing.

My sincere appreciation goes to Katt Lowe for not only rekindling my passion for Eastern medicine and metaphysical studies but also for imparting the invaluable wisdom of using my senses to detect stagnation within the body's Chi system, enabling me to focus and create from the depths of my heart.

Lastly, I want to extend my sincere gratitude and thanks to Michele Guzy for giving me the confidence and courage to bring this book to life.

Together, we can continue to transform lives and promote holistic wellbeing. Thank you.

— **Dr. Tracy Rosa**

CONTENTS

06
HOW THE LYMPH-CHI TREATMENT WORKS 127

07
THYMUS GLAND AND THE DIRECT IMPACT OF LYMPH-CHI TREATMENT .. 153

BACKGROUND AND JOURNEY TO CREATING THE LYMPH-CHI TREATMENT

Thank you for joining me on this journey toward holistic healthcare. I'm Dr. Tracy Rosa, excited to share my knowledge and experience. Throughout my career, I've dedicated myself to studying and practicing a variety of healing modalities, including acupressure, advanced bodywork, hypnotherapy energy medicine, and the metaphysical body. My passion lies in helping individuals achieve wellness in every aspect of their lives.

I've dedicated the last 15 years to exploring an integrative and evidence-based approach to healthcare. My unique approach combines Eastern and Western medicine, diving into the intricate details of how these approaches can complement each other to create optimal health outcomes. We can achieve true healing and wellbeing by treating the whole person—mind, body, brain, soul, and spirit.

I bring a unique perspective as a metaphysician, licensed massage professional, clinical hypnotherapist, Reiki master, and hands-on healing spiritual minister. I understand the importance of addressing the metaphysical aspects of an individual's health, such as their thoughts, emotions, and energy. By combining this approach with advanced bodywork and hypnotherapy, I can offer a comprehensive approach to healing.

My goal has always been to help my clients achieve optimal physical, mental, emotional, and spiritual wellbeing. I've seen the power of integrative medicine firsthand, and I'm excited to share my knowledge and experience with you. I hope this book will inspire you to take control of your health and explore holistic healing possibilities. Together, we can create a new path toward optimal health and wellbeing.

Over the years, I have personally experienced the transformative power of Eastern medicine in treating a wide range of conditions, including chronic pain, stress, post-op surgery, and injuries. At the same time, I was also interested in the latest research and findings from Western medicine, particularly in terms of the lymphatic system and the different treatments offered for healing, as well as its role in maintaining a healthy immune system. I wondered whether there was a way to combine both principles with the latest scientific knowledge to create a more effective and holistic approach to health and wellness.

Through years of research and practice, I developed the Lymph-Chi Treatment. This treatment uses gentle touch, breath work, and visualization to stimulate the lymphatic system and promote the natural flow of lymphatic fluids throughout the body. This improves the immune system and aids in the removal of toxins, as well as swelling and inflammation. The energy work also assists in removing mental and emotional blocks that could worsen the condition.

By combining the strengths of both Eastern and Western medicine, everyone can benefit from their respective approaches. For example, Western medicine focuses on treating symptoms, while Eastern medicine looks at the root cause of the problem. Western medicine is known for its advanced technology and diagnostic tools, while Eastern medicine emphasizes natural remedies and preventative care. So, I developed a new approach to healing that was more effective than either approach on its own. I am now dedicated to sharing this approach with others and helping them achieve optimal physical, mental, emotional, and spiritual wellbeing. I understand that as complex beings, a holistic approach is needed to address all aspects of our health.

I also believe that incorporating metaphysical healing is crucial in achieving optimal health and wellness. As a certified clinical hypnotherapist, I understand the power of the mind in achieving physical healing. By addressing negative thoughts and beliefs, I can release emotional and psychological stress, which can contribute to physical dysfunction. Metaphysical healing recognizes that we each have an energy system, and that disruptions or imbalances in this system can lead to physical, mental, or emotional distress. By addressing the metaphysical aspects of ourselves, such as our thoughts, emotions, and beliefs, we can achieve physical healing and overall wellness.

I am passionate about sharing my journey and expertise with you, revealing how I've created a unique, integrative, evidence-based approach to healing and fostering mental and physical wellbeing. My ultimate goal with my work is to bridge the gap between these two branches of healthcare and bring them together as allies to provide the best possible care.

The Covid-19 pandemic has highlighted the need for a revolutionary new approach to healthcare. We've seen firsthand how the traditional medical system, while essential in many ways, has its flaws and limitations. We need a new approach that focuses on the root causes of illness and seeks to achieve true healing by addressing the whole person, not just the physical symptoms.

Through my journey and expertise, I'll guide you through incorporating Eastern and Western medicine and metaphysical healing into your own life. Together, we'll explore the connection between the mind, brain, body, soul, and spirit, and how we can achieve true balance and wellness in all our lives.

I'm excited to help you release the limitations of your past, stretch your tolerance for what arises in the present, and foster hope for the future. By treating Eastern and Western medicine as allies and partners, we can create a new path toward optimal physical, mental, emotional, and spiritual wellbeing.

PURPOSE OF THE BOOK

In this book, I will take you through the Lymph-Chi Treatment, exploring how it works, the roots of Chi in Traditional Chinese Medicine, and the latest scientific research supporting its efficacy. We will delve into the intricate connections between the lymphatic system and the body's energy systems, exploring how blockages in Chi can impact lymphatic function and lead to various physical, emotional, and mental health issues.

In the following pages, you will learn more about the treatment and its potential to transform your health and wellness. You will discover how this groundbreaking approach can help you achieve greater vitality, resilience, and rebalance in all aspects of your life.

Finally, I will share with you the techniques and approaches I have developed to rebalance the mind-body-brain-spirit-soul connection and optimize lymphatic function, as well as the many success stories of clients who have experienced the transformative power of this treatment. By the end of this book, you will deeply understand the Lymph-Chi Treatment and how it can help you achieve optimal health and wellness.

THE LYMPH-CHI TREATMENT AT A GLANCE

Welcome to the world of Lymph-Chi Treatment, a ground-breaking approach to health and wellness that blends the best of Eastern energy medicine with the latest research results from Western medical science.

But what is the Lymph-Chi Treatment?

This is a revolutionary approach to health and wellness that I have developed over my 15 years of practice. At its core, this treatment is based on the idea that the body's energy systems, particularly the flow of Chi, according to Eastern medical practice, can be harnessed to optimize lymphatic function, leading to improved health and wellness. With the potential to transform the way we think about our bodies and our health, this approach represents a new paradigm in integrating Eastern and Western medicine, combining ancient wisdom with the latest scientific research on the lymphatic system.

At the heart of this approach is the Eastern medical principle of Chi, the highly effective and essential energy that flows through the body's meridian channels. These meridians are like highways that carry energy and information to every part of the body. The Lymph-Chi Treatment uses the meridians in the body by applying gentle pressure on specific acupuncture points to alleviate dysfunctions that lead to physical and mental discomforts. This treatment does not involve needles or breaking the skin. A disruption or obstruction in the Chi's flow may result in imbalances and disease. By combining the principles of Eastern medicine with a deep understanding of the lymphatic system, the Lymph-Chi treatment aims to restore balance and promote overall healing for the mind, brain, body, soul, and spirit. Using this concept as a foundation, I have developed techniques that enable me to work with clients to identify and unblock areas in which energy is stagnant, helping restore the body's natural flow of energy.

Ultimately, the Lymph-Chi represents an innovative approach to health and wellness that draws on the best of both Eastern and Western medical traditions to help clients achieve optimal lymphatic health and overall wellness of the body. Research rooted in Western medicine has also helped refine our understanding of how the lymphatic system works, and I have incorporated this knowledge into my approach into different lymphatic treatments. The lymphatic system is essential to the body's immunological response and aids in the elimination of toxins as well as other wastes. It is also a crucial part of the circulatory system, as it helps move fluids throughout the body, keeping our organs and tissues healthy. By combining Eastern and Western approaches, and through this treatment, clients can take control of their health, allowing them to experience various benefits, both short-term and long-term.

These benefits can include improved breathing and sleep quality. Clients also report quicker healing times after surgery or injury when they undergo Lymph-Chi Treatment, as the techniques used in the treatment help reduce inflammation and promote the body's natural healing response. Beyond its physical benefits, Lymph-Chi Treatment has a significant effect on an individual's mental and emotional health. Restoring a healthy flow of Chi and lymph fluids may help people feel less stressed and anxious, sleep better, and have improved overall moods and cognitive abilities, helping to create a deep sense of relaxation and rejuvenation, to restore the mind-brain-body-spirit-soul connection that is so essential for optimal wellbeing.

As mentioned earlier, the lymphatic system is an intricate web of organs and veins that is essential to preserving health. It removes waste and toxins from the body and fights infections and diseases. When the lymphatic system is compromised, it can lead to various health problems, from swelling and inflammation to chronic fatigue and even autoimmune disorders. But through lighter touch, a lighter pumping motion to direct the fluid, stretching, and acupressure in specific areas, Lymph-Chi will help stimulate the flow of the lymphatic system, moving any stagnant Chi/energy blockages through the meridian channels. This promotes the optimal functioning of the lymphatic system and helps prevent and treat a wide range of health problems.

BENEFITS OF THE LYMPH-CHI TREATMENT

This treatment offers a range of benefits that can improve the overall health and wellness of individuals who follow the treatment approach, as briefly outlined in the previous section. In more detail, these benefits include the following:

Improved Lymphatic Function

The healthiness of a human body highly depends on the circulatory system, of Which the lymphatic system is an essential component. It cleanses the body of waste and toxins, wards off illness and infections, and maintains fluid balance. Several health issues, including edema, irritation, and fluid retention, may result from the lymphatic system not operating at its best. The Lymphatic-Chi Treatment can address these issues through a variety of techniques, including acupressure, stretching, and pumping, allowing toxins to be efficiently eliminated from the body.

Moreover, the Lymph-Chi Treatment can help you maintain a healthy weight, lowering the chances of developing obesity-related diseases like coronary artery disease, Type 2 diabetes, and high blood pressure by decreasing the level of fluid in the body and improving overall body composition.

Enhanced Energy Flow to Reduce Stress and Anxiety

The Lymph-Chi Treatment employs an integrated principle of both Eastern and Western medicine practices to unblock meridians and improve the flow of Chi throughout the body. This may lead to an improvement in energy flow and foster a feeling of vigor and wellbeing. Some clients who have tried this approach for rejuvenation have testified to feeling more energized, focused, and alert, with improved overall vitality.

Stress and anxiety can lead to physical and emotional exhaustion, negatively impacting our overall health and wellness. Lymph-Chi can help in lowering stress, anxiety, and sadness by improving energy flow, all while promoting relaxation and calmness by unblocking the channels and meridians that carry vital energy through the body.

This treatment, which works to improve energy flow, also helps reduce stress hormone levels, such as cortisol. When cortisol levels are elevated, it can cause a range of health problems, including high blood pressure, weight gain, and an increased risk of heart disease.

Lymph-Chi Treatment can help decrease the body's stress response, which can improve sleep quality, reduce muscle tension, and improve overall wellbeing.

Also, the Lymph-Chi Treatment helps in promoting mental healthiness. By promoting relaxation and calmness, the technique can help limit symptoms of anxiety and depression. It can also help increase focus, concentration, and mental clarity, allowing individuals to manage stress better and improve their overall quality of life.

Faster Healing

When the body is injured, it is also the duty of the lymphatic system to ensure that the injured cells and tissues are healed and as fast as possible. In the same vein, the system also helps remove damaged tissue, reduce inflammation, and bring immune cells to the site of injury to help fight infection.

However, if the lymphatic system isn't working at its best, this process can be stalled, leading to prolonged healing times and an increased risk of infection.

The Lymph-Chi Treatment has been shown to speed up the healing process by boosting the function of the lymphatic system and optimizing the flow of Chi in the body. By removing excess fluids and toxins from the area of injury, the body can better repair damaged tissues and restore function. Additionally, by reducing inflammation, the Lymph-Chi treatment can help minimize pain and discomfort during the healing process.

From first-hand experience, the Lymph-Chi Treatment has been seen to improve post-operative recovery times. By promoting optimal lymphatic function, this will help clients see improvement in their recovery process by noticing reduced swelling and discomfort, leading to a faster return to normal activities.

Improved Breathing Patterns

In addition to promoting the lymphatic fluid that carries the toxins and stagnation to drain, the Lymph-Chi Treatment can also help improve breathing patterns. This is achieved by unblocking the meridians and channels associated with the respiratory system. By promoting the flow of Chi and reducing fluid retention in the lungs, the Lymph-Chi Treatment can be particularly beneficial for individuals with respiratory conditions, such as asthma or chronic obstructive pulmonary disease (COPD).

Both asthma and COPD have been associated with inflammation and airway constriction, which can make breathing difficult. Clients with these complications can exhibit symptoms of wheezing, coughing, and shortness of breath.

People with asthma who received any type of lymphatic treatment experienced significant improvements in lung function and reduced symptoms like coughing and wheezing. The same applies to people with COPD who have formally received treatments for improvements in lung function, exercise capacity, and quality of life, meaning we can associate such benefits to Lymph-Chi Treatment.

Improved breathing patterns can also lead to improved sleep, as individuals with respiratory conditions may experience interruptions in their sleep due to difficulty breathing. By improving lung function and reducing inflammation, the Lymph-Chi Treatment can help promote restful sleep and overall wellbeing.

Rebalancing The Mind-Brain-Body-Spirit-Soul

The Lymph-Chi Treatment recognizes that the body's health is interconnected with the mind, spirit, and soul's health. Improving lymphatic function and promoting energy flow can help create a sense of harmony between these aspects of the self.

The Lymph-Chi Treatment can also help release emotional blockages that may impact overall health and wellbeing. You should feel more relaxed, centered, and grounded through targeted lighter touch, stretching, a lighter pumping motion to direct the fluid, and acupressure. This can lead to improved mental clarity, reduced stress and anxiety, and greater inner peace.

Furthermore, the Lymph-Chi Treatment can help individuals connect with their more profound sense of purpose and meaning in life.

It offers a holistic approach to health and wellbeing that recognizes the interconnection between the mind, body, brain, spirit, and soul. By promoting lymphatic function and energy flow, this treatment can help individuals achieve optimal health and wellness on all levels.

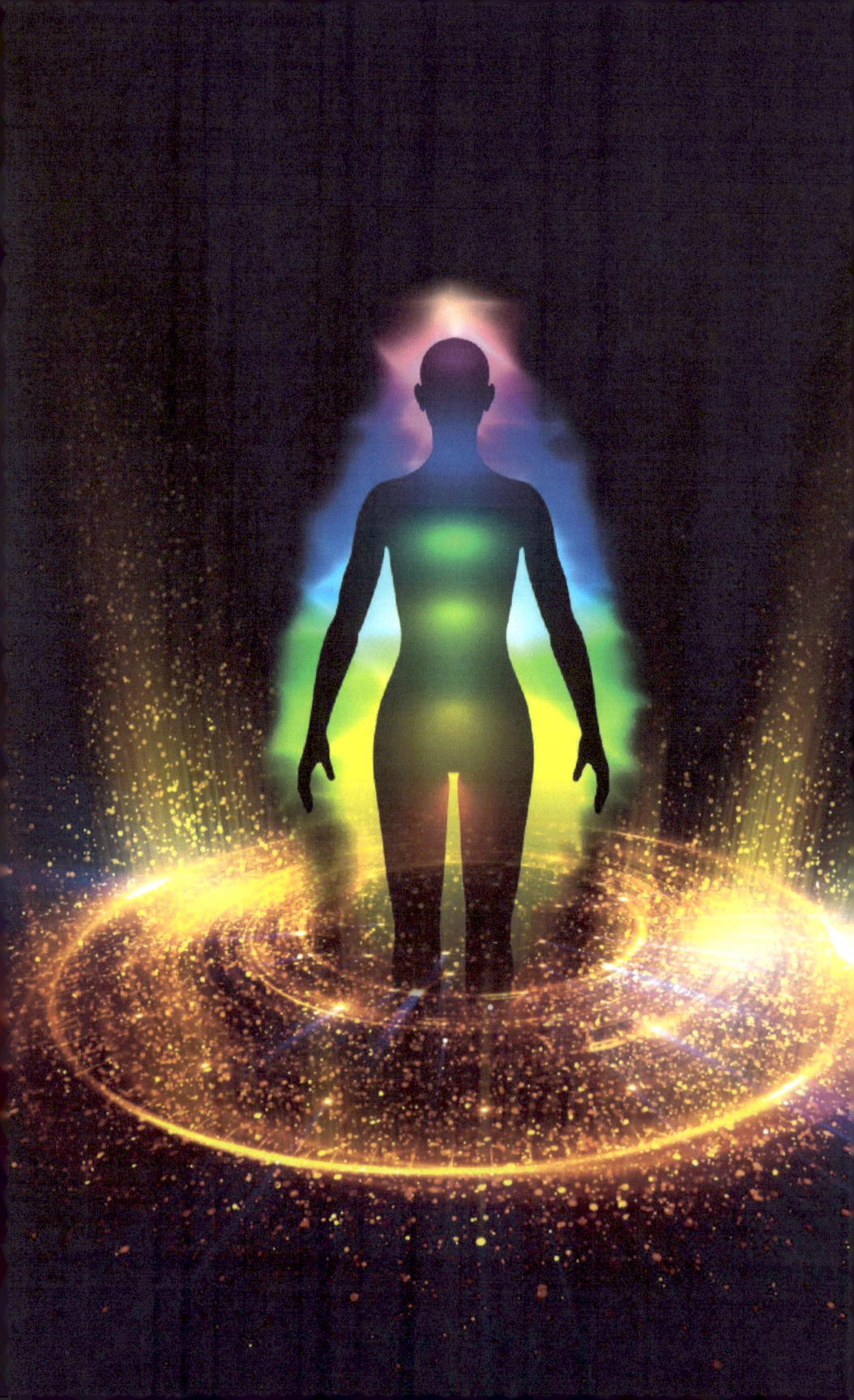

UNDERSTANDING CHI AND EASTERN MEDICINE

Energy is essential to our overall health and wellbeing and is critical in supporting lymphatic health and post-operative recovery. The lymphatic system removes waste and toxins from the body, and energy is required to support its proper functioning.

This section will explore the ancient Eastern concept of Chi, which is believed to be the vital energy that flows through the body and supports various bodily functions, including the lymphatic system. We will delve into the 14 meridian channels through which Chi flows and how it interacts with each organ and system in the body.

Furthermore, we will examine the lineage of the Chi system beliefs and its integration into other practices, such as Tai Chi, Qigong, and acupuncture, which have been shown to support lymphatic health and post-operative recovery. We will also discuss the meditative state, its effects on Chi, and the connection between Chi and the nervous system.

By the end of this section, you will better understand energy's critical role in supporting lymphatic health and post-operative recovery. So, let's explore the fascinating world of Chi and Eastern medicine together.

What is Chi According to Eastern Medicine?

In Eastern medicine, Chi is the foundation of good health and wellbeing. According to Eastern medicine philosophy, everything in the universe is composed of energy, including the human body. Therefore, the flow of Chi is essential for maintaining the balance of this energy and promoting overall health.

The concept of Chi is not unique to Traditional Chinese Medicine (TCM); it is present in many other ancient Eastern practices, as well, such as Ayurveda, yoga, and Buddhism. Chi is thought to be the force that animates the body and keeps it alive. It is believed to be present in all living things, including animals, plants, and the environment. The flow of Chi is considered to be fundamental to good health and vitality.

Eastern medicine views the human body as a complex system of interconnected channels or meridians through which Chi flows. These channels form a network that connects the various organs and systems in the body, allowing them to work together in harmony. Each meridian is associated with specific organs and functions, and Chi is said to circulate through them, nourishing and supporting the body's various functions.

The flow of Chi through the 14 main channels that the meridian system is divided into can be influenced by many things, including emotions, diet, lifestyle, and environmental factors. When the flow of Chi is disrupted or blocked, it can lead to imbalances in the body, resulting in illness and disease. With the application of Lymph-Chi Treatment, one of the aims is to restore balance to the body by identifying and addressing these imbalances through a range of modalities, including herbal medicine and nutritional therapy.

An imbalance or blockage in the flow of Chi is believed to be the root cause of many health problems. By restoring the proper flow of Chi, we promote our overall health and wellness and prevent illness and disease.

There are two primary types of Chi: Original Chi and Acquired Chi.

Original Chi is the energy we inherit from our parents and is said to reside in the kidneys. It provides the foundation for our overall health and vitality.

Acquired Chi, on the other hand, is the energy we absorb from our environment and is influenced by our lifestyle, diet, and other external factors.

In addition to the two primary types of Chi, there are also specific qualities associated with Chi in general, including Yin and Yang. Yin Chi is the more passive, feminine energy associated with calmness, intuition, and creativity, whereas Yang Chi is the more active, masculine energy associated with qualities such as strength, assertiveness, and action. But we will discuss the Yin and Yang organs further in the coming chapters, detailing how their care can help retain optimal health.

In summary, Chi is the fundamental essence of life. It is critical to helping the body's functions and promote overall health and wellbeing. Understanding Chi and its importance is essential to Eastern medicine and can provide valuable insights into alternative approaches to health and wellness.

The Lineage of the Chi System Beliefs

The Chi system is a belief system that dates back thousands of years in Chinese history. Its roots can be traced back to the ancient Chinese belief that the universe is made up of energy, known as Chi, which flows through all living beings and their environment. The belief in Chi has been a fundamental aspect of Traditional Chinese Medicine, martial arts, and Taoist philosophy.

According to the Chi belief system, the human body has two main sources of Chi. The first source is the Chi inherited from our parents at birth, known as ancestral Chi. The second source is the Chi we acquire from the food we eat, the air we breathe, and the environment around us. This acquired Chi is known as environmental Chi.

The lineage of the Chi system beliefs is deeply rooted in the history of China, dating back to the legendary Yellow Emperor, Huangdi, who is considered the father of Chinese medicine. Huangdi is believed to have lived in China around 2600 B.C. and is said to have written the Huangdi Neijing, also known as *The Yellow Emperor's Classic of Internal Medicine.*

The Huangdi Neijing is a fundamental text of Traditional Chinese Medicine, and it is still studied and revered by practitioners of TCM today. The text is divided into the Suwen (Basic Questions) and the Lingshu (Miraculous Pivot). The Suwen describes the fundamental principles of TCM, including the flow of Chi and its relationship with the internal organs and bodily systems. The Lingshu focuses on the application of moxibustion techniques.

According to TCM philosophy, the body is a complex network of meridians or channels through which vital energy or Chi flows. This energy is believed to be responsible for maintaining physical and emotional health, and when it becomes blocked or disrupted, it can lead to illness or disease. The Huangdi Neijing describes the flow of Chi and how it relates to the internal organs, bodily systems, and emotions, providing a foundation for TCM diagnosis and treatment.

Over the centuries, the principles of TCM have been passed down through various lineages and schools of thought, each adding its insights and techniques. Today, TCM is a diverse and dynamic field, encompassing many practices, including herbal medicine, massage, nutritional therapy, and exercise, all aimed at restoring balance and harmony to the body and mind.

Over time, the Chinese developed various forms of martial arts, such as Tai Chi and Qigong, which incorporated the principles of the Chi system. These practices focused on cultivating and manipulating Chi to improve health, strength, and overall wellbeing.

In modern times, the Chi system beliefs have become more widely accepted and are practiced worldwide. Many people use techniques, such as Tai Chi, to improve their health and wellbeing. While the scientific basis for the Chi system is still debated, its principles and practices have proven to be effective for many people over thousands of years.

How Essential is the Chi Energy?

Life is dependent on the flow of Chi. This rule is crucial for the following reasons:

For our wellbeing: For health and wellness to exist, there must be the opportunity for Chi to flow freely. There is no pain when there is free flow, according to The Yellow Emperor's Classic of Internal Medicine (237 B.C.). This means that no free flow exists in places of anguish. The guiding idea of Chinese medicine is to encourage the free flow of Chi and blood.

Regarding our surroundings: The goal of feng shui, both an art and a science, is to create an atmosphere in which Chi can flow freely. Depending on the type of Chi in your surroundings, it may either feed or drain your life energy.

With regard to nature: Qigong and other meditative mind-body exercises can be used to harness Chi, which is present in all living things. Utilizing Chi involves living in harmony with the seasons, eating locally grown food, sleeping at night, and waking up in the morning to maintain a healthy sleep-wake cycle.

The 14 Meridian Channels and How Chi Flows Through the Body

The meridian system is the network of channels through which Chi flows, connecting the various organs and systems in the body. There are 14 main meridians in the body, with each channel associated with a specific organ or system. The flow of Chi through these channels is essential for maintaining good health and wellbeing.

The 14 meridians are divided into two categories, the Yin meridians, and the Yang meridians. The Yin meridians are associated with the body's interior and are responsible for nourishing and cooling the body. The Yang meridians, on the other hand, are related to the body's exterior and are responsible for warming and protecting the body.

The 14 meridian channels in the body include:

- Lung Meridian
- Large Intestine Meridian
- Stomach Meridian
- Spleen Meridian
- Heart Meridian
- Small Intestine Meridian
- Bladder Meridian
- Kidney Meridian
- Pericardium Meridian
- Triple Burner Meridian
- Gallbladder Meridian
- Liver Meridian
- Governing Vessel Meridian

- Conception Vessel Meridian

The meridian system is also interconnected, with each channel affecting and influencing the others. Chi flows through these channels in a specific order, and each channel has a time of day when its energy is at its peak. For example, if a client is experiencing respiratory issues, the lung meridian channel or other modalities can be used to restore the flow of Chi to this area. Chi also flows through the meridians in a cyclical pattern, which is known as the circadian rhythm of Chi flow. For instance, the lung meridian's energy is at its peak from 3-5 am, while the large intestine meridian's energy is at its peak from 5-7 am. An imbalance in one channel can lead to imbalances in others, so it is essential to take a holistic approach when diagnosing and treating energy imbalances in the body.

The 24-Hour Chi Cycle

In Traditional Chinese Medicine, it is believed that the flow of Qi or Chi follows a specific sequence throughout the body, circulating from one organ to another. Additionally, each channel or meridian that the Qi flows through has a specific two-hour "high tide" period each day. This sequence of high tide includes:

- Liver =>1-3 a.m.
- Lungs => 3-5 a.m.
- Large Intestines => 5-7 a.m.
- Stomach => 7-9 a.m.
- Spleen => 9-11 a.m.
- Heart => 11 a.m.-1 p.m.
- Small Intestines => 1-3 p.m.
- Bladder => 3-5 p.m.
- Kidneys => 5-7 p.m.
- Pericardium => 7-9 p.m.

- Triple Warmer => 9-11 p.m.
- Gall Bladder => 11 p.m.-1 a.m.

After the sequence is complete, it repeats, beginning with the lungs. This 24-hour cycle of the Chi flow is thought to significantly impact the health and functioning of the body's organs and systems. By understanding and working with this cycle, TCM practitioners aim to optimize the flow of Qi and promote overall health and wellbeing.

Yin and Yang of Organs in the Body

As we've previously discussed, the body contains a network of channels called meridians that transport energy, or Chi, throughout the body. These meridians are connected to various organs and systems, classified as either Yin or Yang.

Yin and Yang are complementary principles, representing the harmony of opposite natural forces. Yin is associated with cold, quiet, and restful qualities, while Yang is associated with heat, activity, and movement. In the body, Yin organs are those that store vital substances and energy, while Yang organs are those that generate and transform energy.

There are five Yin and five Yang organs in the body, and they are paired based on their complementary functions. The Yin organs are the heart, lungs, spleen, kidneys, and liver, while the Yang organs are the small intestine, large intestine, stomach, bladder, and gallbladder. These organs communicate with each other through the meridians, and any imbalance or disharmony in one organ can affect the function of its paired organ. The five Yin and five Yang organs are paired based on their complementary functions, which is essential for optimal function of the lymphatic system and the body in general. The Yin organs produce, store, and regulate vital substances, such as blood, fluids, and essence. In contrast, the Yang organs are responsible for processing and eliminating waste and excess materials from the body.

For instance, the lungs, as a Yin organ, are responsible for taking in air and distributing oxygen throughout the body. They work in harmony with the large intestine, a Yang organ that eliminates waste and toxins from the body. If the lungs are compromised, the large intestine may become affected and cease to function properly, leading to constipation or other digestive problems. Similarly, if the large intestine is not working properly, it can affect the lungs' ability to take in oxygen, leading to respiratory issues, such as shortness of breath.

For example, the liver and gallbladder are paired organs, with the liver being the Yin organ and the gallbladder being the Yang organ. The liver is responsible for storing and regulating blood, while the gallbladder is responsible for storing and secreting bile to aid digestion. If the liver isn't balanced, it can affect the gallbladder's function, leading to digestive problems, such as gallstones or indigestion. Similarly, if the gallbladder isn't in proper alignment, it can affect another important part of the body, such as the liver, and lead to irritability or anger.

How Yin and Yang Organs Communicate

The organs communicate through the meridians, and the flow of energy and blood through these channels is essential to maintain their harmonious function. The meridian system is often described as a network of interdependent channels through which vital energy, or Chi, flows. Each meridian is associated with a particular organ system, and the flow of Chi through each meridian is believed to be influenced by the health and function of the associated organ. However, meridians are not isolated entities; they are interconnected with one another in various ways.

That being said, disruptions to the flow of Chi in one meridian can impact the flow of Chi in other meridians. For example, suppose there is a blockage in the flow of Chi in the stomach meridian. In that case, it can affect the spleen meridian, leading to symptoms like fatigue, poor digestion, and weakened immunity.

Similarly, suppose there is an imbalance in the flow of Chi in the liver meridian. In that case, it can affect the gallbladder meridian, leading to symptoms like pain in the ribs and shoulders and digestive issues.

Therefore, the meridian system is seen as an interconnected web, where the health and function of one meridian can impact the health and function of other meridians. This is why taking a holistic approach to health is important, focusing on the balance and flow of Chi throughout the body rather than just treating individual symptoms or conditions.

The goal of treatment is to restore balance and harmony to the body's Yin and Yang organs and their associated meridians. This can be accomplished through various modalities, including acupuncture, herbal medicine, dietary therapy, and Qigong. By addressing imbalances and promoting the smooth flow of Chi, clients can experience improved health and wellbeing.

Ultimately, people who live their life in alignment with the principles of Yin and Yang and Chi experience an inner calmness and focused presence. In Eastern medicine, this state is called good shen, which means heart Chi. So, if you can attain this level, you can possess a vitality and life force that is reflected in your eyes. This allows you to remain composed and tranquil, giving your undivided attention to the task at hand. This also emanates a vibrant positive energy, enveloping individuals in expansive energy fields that facilitate their rapid recovery from both stressful situations and interactions with others.

Chi's Association with Each Organ and System in The Body

According to Eastern medical practice, Chi is believed to be present in all living things. It flows through the body's 14 meridian channels associated with specific organs and systems. Each organ and system in the body is connected to a meridian channel, and the flow of Chi through these channels is essential for maintaining the balance and health of each organ and system.

Here are some examples of Chi's association with each organ and system in the body:

Lung: The lung meridian channel is the first line of defense against external pathogens that can cause illness. It is associated with the respiratory system and is crucial in maintaining healthy lung function, including oxygen circulation throughout the body. The lung meridian channel is also believed to be associated with the skin, which is considered a protective barrier against external pathogens.

The lung meridian channel is responsible for the immune system's proper functioning, which helps fight off infections and diseases. It is believed to be closely connected to the body's ability to generate Chi, vital energy necessary for maintaining good health and preventing illness.

Imbalances in the lung meridian channel can result in various health problems, including respiratory issues, such as asthma and bronchitis, allergies, colds, and the flu. In addition, the lung meridian channel is believed to be connected to emotional health, with imbalances in this channel potentially leading to anxiety, grief, and sadness.

Various techniques, including herbal remedies and lifestyle changes, can help balance the lung meridian channel. These treatments aim to restore the flow of Chi through the lung meridian channel, promoting healthy lung function, boosting immunity, and supporting overall physical and emotional wellbeing.

Large Intestine: The large intestine meridian channel is considered one of the digestive system's primary channels. This channel starts at the tip of the index finger, moves up the arm, over the shoulder, and down the side of the body, eventually ending at the nostril.

The large intestine meridian channel plays a crucial role in the body's ability to eliminate waste and toxins. It is responsible for transporting waste products from the colon and rectum to the outside of the body. In addition to waste removal, the large intestine meridian channel also helps to regulate the body's fluid balance, playing an important role in preventing constipation and maintaining regular bowel movements.

It is believed to be closely connected to the lung meridian channel. This connection is because the lungs are responsible for taking in oxygen and eliminating carbon dioxide, much like how the large intestine meridian channel eliminates waste from the body. Proper functioning of the large intestine meridian channel is important for overall digestive health and maintaining a healthy immune system.

Stomach: The stomach meridian channel in Traditional Chinese Medicine is believed to be one of the most important meridians in the body. It is responsible for the proper digestion and absorption of nutrients from our food. According to TCM, the stomach meridian channel starts from the face, specifically the cheekbone, and runs down the body's front surface, passing through the chest and abdomen and ending at the foot's second toe.

It is responsible for breaking down food and sending it to the Small Intestine for further processing. When the stomach meridian channel is not functioning correctly, it can lead to various digestive issues, such as bloating, indigestion, and constipation. The stomach meridian channel's function is to extract nutrients from food and distribute them throughout the body, so a blockage or disturbance in this channel can lead to malnourishment and weakness.

The stomach meridian channel is closely related to the Earth element and is affected by external factors, such as humidity and dampness. Thus, excessive consumption of cold, raw, and damp foods like salads and smoothies can lead to an imbalance in the stomach meridian channel and affect its proper functioning.

Acupuncture, acupressure, and other TCM therapies can help restore balance to the stomach meridian channel and improve digestive health. Along with these therapies, incorporating warm, cooked foods and avoiding excessive consumption of cold, raw, and damp foods can help maintain the proper functioning of the stomach meridian channel and ensure the efficient digestion and absorption of nutrients from the food we eat.

Spleen: The spleen meridian channel is not only associated with the digestive system but also plays an essential role in the immune system by producing white blood cells. The spleen is responsible for transforming food into nutrients and transporting those nutrients to the rest of the body. It also controls the movement of fluids in the body, particularly the transformation of fluids into Qi, which is then circulated throughout the body.

When the spleen meridian channel functions correctly, it promotes healthy digestion and absorption of nutrients, maintains proper fluid balance, and supports a healthy immune system. However, when the spleen meridian channel is imbalanced or blocked, it can lead to unfavorable symptoms, such as abdominal bloating, diarrhea, fatigue, and weakened immune function.

Heart: The heart meridian channel is a crucial part of the circulatory system and is responsible for pumping blood. The heart is believed to be the center of one's being, responsible for emotions, thoughts, and consciousness. The heart meridian channel starts at the heart and runs down the arm, ending at the pinky finger.

The heart meridian channel is responsible for pumping blood, regulating blood pressure, and maintaining a healthy heart rhythm. A healthy heart meridian channel ensures that the heart is functioning correctly and that there is sufficient blood flow throughout the body. When the heart meridian channel is imbalanced or blocked, it can lead to various heart-related disorders, including palpitations, arrhythmias, and hypertension.

It is also closely related to emotions. The heart is believed to be the organ that governs joy and happiness. So, when the heart meridian channel is imbalanced, it can lead to emotional disturbances, such as anxiety, depression, and insomnia. Balancing the heart's meridian channel is essential to maintaining physical and emotional health.

Small Intestine: The small intestine meridian channel is believed to be associated with the digestive system and plays an important role in the absorption of nutrients from food. The Small Intestine is responsible for breaking down and separating nutrients from the food we eat so that they can be properly absorbed into the bloodstream and transported to other body parts where they are needed.

It starts at the tip of the little finger, runs up the arm and shoulder, and then goes through the heart and chest before ending at the ear. An imbalance in the small intestine meridian channel can lead to digestive problems, such as bloating, gas, and abdominal discomfort. It may also manifest in insomnia, heart palpitations, and anxiety.

To balance and promote the proper flow of Chi through the small intestine meridian channel, acupuncture or acupressure techniques can be used to stimulate specific points along the channel. Nutritional and lifestyle changes, as well as herbal remedies, are recommended to support digestive health and overall wellbeing.

Bladder: The bladder meridian channel is believed to be one of the body's longest and most complex meridians. It is associated with the urinary system and removes waste and excess bodily fluid. The bladder meridian begins at the inner corner of the eye, runs over the forehead, and zigzags over the scalp before descending the neck, back, and legs.

The bladder is seen as more than just a physical organ that eliminates waste. It is believed to be connected to the body's ability to adapt to change and maintain balance. The bladder meridian is thought to help regulate the body's fluids, which is crucial for proper kidney function and overall health.

Imbalances in the bladder meridian can result in various symptoms, including urinary tract infections, bladder inflammation, and even emotional stress. Acupuncture or herbal remedies help balance the bladder meridian and improve overall health. For example, acupuncture points along the bladder meridian on the back can help to relieve lower back pain, while points on the leg can help alleviate urinary problems.

Kidney: This meridian channel is considered one of the most important channels in the body as it is associated with the foundation of Yin and Yang, the two complementary energies crucial for maintaining health and balance. The kidney meridian channel regulates the body's water metabolism and electrolyte balance, crucial in controlling blood pressure.

The kidney meridian channel is also associated with the reproductive system and is believed to be the source of sexual energy, essential for reproductive health and overall vitality. The kidney meridian channel is also associated with the endocrine system, which regulates the body's hormones, including cortisol.

Imbalances in this meridian channel can lead to various health problems, including urinary and reproductive issues, fatigue, lower back pain, and even depression.

Pericardium: The pericardium meridian channel is the "heart protector" meridian. This meridian is associated with the circulatory system and helps regulate the heart's rhythm and protect the heart from emotional stress.

It starts at the chest, runs down the arm's inside, through the palm, and ends at the tip of the middle finger. It is believed to be closely related to the heart meridian channel and is responsible for protecting the heart from emotional disturbances.

When the pericardium meridian is balanced and flowing smoothly, it promotes emotional wellbeing and can help reduce feelings of anxiety and stress. However, an imbalance or blockage in the pericardium meridian can lead to emotional instability and heart-related issues, such as palpitations or chest pain.

To promote the health of the pericardium meridian, recommended treatments include acupuncture, herbal medicine, nutritional changes, and lifestyle modifications. These treatments aim to restore balance and promote the smooth flow of Chi through the pericardium meridian, which can help support overall heart health and emotional wellbeing.

Triple Burner: The Triple Burner meridian channel is a unique concept not found in Western medicine. It is often described as a "burner" or "heater" that regulates the body's fluids and metabolism. The Triple Burner is considered to be a functional system responsible for regulating the body's fluid balance and temperature and for transforming food into energy.

It consists of three parts, or "burners," corresponding to different body areas. The upper burner is associated with the chest and the respiratory system, the middle burner is associated with the digestive system, and the lower burner is associated with the urinary system and the reproductive organs.

The Triple Burner meridian channel is responsible for energy flow between these three burners. It is believed to be closely connected to the body's metabolism and plays an important role in maintaining fluid balance.

It is considered an important system for maintaining overall health and wellbeing. An imbalance in the Triple Burner can lead to various health problems, including digestive issues, hormonal imbalances, and fluid retention. Maintaining a healthy balance in the Triple Burner is believed to support the body's natural healing processes and promote overall health and vitality.

Gallbladder: The gallbladder meridian channel is an important part of the body's digestive system and is responsible for breaking down fats consumed in the diet. The gallbladder is a small organ that stores bile produced by the liver, which helps our bodies digest fat. The gallbladder meridian channel is responsible for the smooth flow of bile throughout the body and works to ensure that the digestive system functions properly.

When the gallbladder meridian channel is blocked or disrupted, it can lead to problems with digestion, such as nausea, bloating, and diarrhea. Additionally, individuals with a blocked gallbladder meridian channel may experience anger, frustration, or resentment, as these emotions are associated with the gallbladder.

To keep the gallbladder meridian channel healthy and functioning properly, you can engage in activities that promote healthy digestion, such as eating balanced nutrition with plenty of fiber and healthy fats, staying hydrated, and engaging in regular exercise. Acupuncture and acupressure can stimulate the gallbladder meridian channel and promote better digestion. A healthy gallbladder meridian channel is essential for maintaining good digestive health and overall wellbeing.

Liver: The liver meridian channel is associated with the liver and is responsible for the smooth flow of energy, or Chi, throughout the body. The liver is one of the most important organs in the body, responsible for detoxification, hormone production, and regulating metabolism.

The liver stores and regulates the flow of blood and Chi, and the liver meridian channel ensures this flow is smooth and unobstructed. When the liver is healthy and functioning properly, it helps maintain body balance, both physically and emotionally.

The liver meridian channel begins at the big toe and travels up the inside of the leg, through the groin, and up the torso, ending at the rib cage. Along the way, it passes through several important acupuncture points believed to be linked to the liver and its functions.

Some of the common symptoms that are associated with a liver imbalance include fatigue, headaches, dizziness, irritability, and depression. These symptoms can be caused by various factors, including stress, poor diet, alcohol consumption, and exposure to toxins.

There are several ways to support liver health and promote the smooth flow of energy through the liver meridian channel. These may include dietary changes, such as avoiding alcohol and greasy or fatty foods and using acupuncture, acupressure, and herbal remedies. Regular exercise, stress management techniques, and getting enough sleep are also important for maintaining a healthy liver and supporting overall wellbeing.

Governing Vessel: The governing vessel meridian channel, also known as Du Mai in Traditional Chinese Medicine, is one of the eight extraordinary meridians associated with the central nervous system. It runs along the body's midline from the perineum, up through the spine and the back of the neck, ending at the top of the head.

The governing vessel meridian channel regulates the body's energy flow. It is often called the "sea of Yang" because it is a major pathway for the flow of Yang energy in the body. The Yang energy represents the body's active, outward-moving energy that helps drive its various functions.

When the governing vessel meridian channel functions properly, it helps balance and distribute the body's energy throughout all the other meridians, organs, and systems. This can help improve overall health and vitality, enhance mental clarity and focus, and reduce stress and anxiety.

On the other hand, an imbalance or blockage in the governing vessel meridian channel can result in a range of physical and emotional symptoms, including fatigue, poor concentration, headaches, insomnia, and emotional instability.

To help balance and strengthen the governing vessel meridian channel, acupuncture, acupressure, and herbal medicine are often used. Practices such as yoga, Qigong, and meditation can also help promote the flow of energy along this meridian and supporting overall health and wellbeing.

Conception Vessel: The conception vessel, known as the Ren Mai, is one of the eight extraordinary meridians. It is located on the front of the body and runs from the pubic bone to the lower lip. This meridian is associated with the reproductive system and regulates hormones.

In women, the conception vessel is particularly important during pregnancy and Childbirth. It is believed that stimulating certain points along the meridian can help with fertility, regulate menstrual cycles, and alleviate menstrual cramps. Acupuncture or acupressure on this meridian may also help prepare the body for labor and delivery by strengthening the uterus and promoting blood circulation.

In addition to its role in the reproductive system, the conception vessel is also believed to regulate the body's energy flow and promote overall balance and wellbeing. Stimulating certain points along the meridian may help improve digestion, alleviate stress and anxiety, and promote better sleep.

Overall, the conception vessel is a significant meridian in Traditional Chinese Medicine that plays a crucial role in regulating hormonal balance and promoting overall health and wellness. By stimulating specific points along this meridian, practitioners of Traditional Chinese Medicine believe they can help restore balance and harmony to the body, mind, and spirit.

Indications of An Imbalance in Your Chi

The prenatal Chi, or Jing, that we are born with, must last us a lifetime, according to Eastern medicine. This essence is burned, and the lifespan is shortened by behaviors like overworking, stressing out, and abusing the body.

Our neurological system activates the adrenal glands in a flight, fight, or freeze response when stressed. The flow of Chi is interrupted if the body does not swiftly revert to the rest and digest stage. Chi may get stagnated, causing the body as a whole to feel bloated and inflexible. Here are a few indicators that something is wrong with your Chi:

Feeling exhausted most of the time, even when you haven't done much

Feeling tired after a long day or strenuous physical activity is normal. But experiencing exhaustion even when you haven't done much in a day may indicate an imbalance in your Chi.

According to Eastern medicine, when the flow of Chi is disrupted or blocked, the body's natural balance is affected, which can lead to physical and mental fatigue, causing an imbalance in the flow of Chi throughout the body. This can manifest as tiredness, weakness, and lethargy, even when you haven't exerted yourself much. Stress, poor diet, lack of exercise, overwork, or emotional imbalances all contribute to this phenomenon.

You can try practicing Chi-based therapies like acupuncture, acupressure, Tai Chi, Qigong, or meditation to rebalance your Chi and restore your energy levels. These therapies unblock and stimulate the flow of Chi throughout the body, improving circulation and restoring balance to the body's energy systems.

In addition to these therapies, you can make lifestyle changes, such as eating a healthy, balanced diet, getting enough sleep, reducing stress, and incorporating regular exercise into your routine. By caring for your body and mind, you can improve your overall energy levels and achieve a more balanced and harmonious state of being.

Easy weight gain

Easy weight gain can be an indication of an imbalance in your Chi. Traditional Chinese Medicine believes the body is interconnected, with different organ systems and energy channels affecting one another. When the flow of Chi is disrupted or stagnant, it can lead to various health issues, including weight gain.

In TCM, the spleen and liver are the two organs most closely associated with weight management. The spleen is responsible for transforming food into energy, while the liver is responsible for processing and eliminating toxins from the body. If the spleen is weak or the liver is congested, it can create an imbalance in the body's metabolism, causing weight gain.

Excessive weight gain can also be caused by emotional imbalances that affect the flow of Chi. Stress, anxiety, and depression can all cause disruptions in energy flow, leading to weight gain. Emotional eating and a sedentary lifestyle can also contribute to weight gain.

It is important to address the root cause of the imbalance to restore balance to the body and promote healthy weight management. This may involve a combination of dietary changes, exercise, acupuncture, and herbal remedies to support the spleen and liver and improve the flow of Chi. Additionally, addressing emotional imbalances through practices such as meditation, mindfulness, or counseling can also help restore balance to the body and promote healthy weight management.

Prolonged insomnia (this implies that your Yin and Yang are upturned)

Insomnia is a common problem for many people, but it can also indicate an imbalance in your Chi. In Chinese medicine, Yin and Yang are closely tied to sleep and wake cycles. Yin represents the calming, cooling, and restful aspect, while Yang represents the active, warming, and energizing aspect of our bodies.

When the Yin and Yang are upturned, the balance between the two is disrupted. This can cause prolonged insomnia, where you have difficulty falling asleep or staying asleep, leading to fatigue and other health issues.

Several factors, including stress, anxiety, poor nutrition, and lack of exercise can cause an upturned Yin and Yang. To restore balance and improve sleep, it's important to address the root cause of the problem. This may involve incorporating relaxation techniques like meditation or yoga, improving your diet, exercising regularly, and seeking professional help.

If you're experiencing prolonged insomnia, it's essential to seek help from a healthcare practitioner specializing in Eastern medicine or other holistic therapies to help rebalance your Chi and restore restful sleep.

Excess work with little time to allow the body to recover properly

Excess work with little time to allow the body to recover properly can lead to an imbalance in your Chi, causing physical and emotional symptoms. When we overwork and don't give ourselves enough time to rest and recuperate, it can strain our body's energy system.

In Traditional Chinese Medicine, this imbalance is caused by an excess of Yang energy, leading to symptoms like fatigue, irritability, and stress. It can also lead to physical symptoms like muscle tension, headaches, and digestive problems.

To restore balance to your Chi, it's important to take breaks and prioritize rest and self-care. This can include meditation, gentle exercise, and getting enough sleep. It's also important to set boundaries with work and allow yourself time to disconnect and recharge.

By caring for yourself and restoring balance to your Chi, you can prevent further imbalances and support your overall health and wellbeing.

You overindulge in booze and meals with little nutrients

Overindulging in alcohol and meals with little nutrients can lead to an imbalance in your Chi. Alcohol can be taxing on the liver, which is a key organ in Chinese medicine that plays a role in regulating the flow of Chi in the body. Excessive alcohol consumption can result in liver Chi stagnation, which disrupts the body's functions.

Moreover, consuming meals with few nutrients can deplete the body of essential vitamins and minerals necessary for properly functioning the body's systems. When the body is deprived of essential nutrients, it can lead to a weakened immune system, decreased energy levels, and a general feeling of malaise.

An imbalance in the Chi caused by overindulging in alcohol and meals with little nutrients can result in a range of physical and emotional symptoms. These symptoms can include lethargy, mood swings, digestive problems, and skin issues, as well irritability, mood swings, and fatigue. To maintain a healthy balance of Chi, it is important to consume a balanced diet with plenty of nutrient-dense foods and to drink alcohol in moderation.

You are temperamentally irritable and angry, in most cases, with no actual problem

Being temperamentally irritable and angry for no reason can indicate an imbalance in your Chi. In Traditional Chinese Medicine, anger is associated with the liver and its corresponding meridian system. The liver is responsible for the smooth flow of energy in the body, and when this flow is disrupted, it can lead to emotional imbalances.

If you find yourself getting easily agitated and frustrated, even over small matters, it may be a sign that your liver energy is out of balance. This can be caused by stress, overwork, poor diet, lack of exercise, or exposure to toxins.

To address this imbalance, you can focus on supporting your liver and the body's energy flow through practices like acupuncture, Qigong, and Tai Chi. You can also make dietary changes like reducing your intake of alcohol and processed foods and increasing your consumption of fresh fruits and vegetables.

In addition, it may be helpful to identify any sources of stress in your life and take steps to manage them. This could involve practicing mindfulness meditation, taking breaks throughout the day to relax and de-stress, or seeking support from a therapist or counselor.

Remember, an imbalanced Chi can manifest in various physical, emotional, and mental symptoms. You can promote overall health and wellbeing by paying attention to your body and taking steps to address any imbalances.

Irregular menstrual cycle

An irregular menstrual cycle can indicate an imbalance in one's Chi. In Traditional Chinese Medicine, the menstrual cycle reflects the body's overall health and balance of energies. When the body's Chi is out of balance, it can manifest in various ways, including changes in the menstrual cycle.

An irregular menstrual cycle can indicate a deficiency or excess of Yin or Yang energies in the body. In TCM, the Yin energy is associated with the female reproductive system and the blood, while the Yang energy is associated with the male reproductive system and the sperm. An excess of Yang energy can cause the menstrual cycle to become shorter and heavier, while a deficiency of Yin energy can cause it to become longer and lighter.

Other factors contributing to an irregular menstrual cycle include stress, poor diet, lack of exercise, and hormonal imbalances. It is important to seek the advice of a qualified TCM practitioner to determine the underlying cause of the imbalance and develop a treatment plan that includes acupuncture, herbal medicine, dietary and lifestyle changes, and other Chi-based therapies. By addressing the root cause of the imbalance, it is possible to restore the body's natural balance and promote regularity in the menstrual cycle.

Your body hurts and aches

Frequently experiencing pain and discomfort in your body may be indicative of an imbalance in your Chi. The smooth flow of Chi throughout the body is essential to maintaining physical, mental, and emotional wellbeing.

An imbalance in your Chi can cause stagnation or blockages in the energy flow, leading to pain and discomfort in the affected area. This pain can manifest as headaches, joint pain, muscle aches, or bodily discomfort.

Many factors can contribute to an imbalance in your Chi, such as stress, poor diet, lack of exercise, and environmental toxins. Addressing the underlying cause of the imbalance and working to restore the flow of Chi can help alleviate these symptoms.

Practices like acupressure, Tai Chi, and Qigong are all designed to help balance and restore the flow of Chi in the body. These techniques can help stimulate the body's natural healing processes, reduce pain and inflammation, and promote overall wellbeing.

It is important to note that a medical professional should always evaluate and treat chronic or severe pain. However, incorporating Chi-based therapies into your wellness routine can help address underlying imbalances and promote optimal health and vitality.

Meditative State and Effects on Chi

In Traditional Chinese Medicine, the concept of Chi is closely linked to meditation. Meditation is believed to help regulate the flow of Chi through the body, promoting balance and healing.

Meditation is a practice that has been around for thousands of years and is used by many cultures worldwide as a means of spiritual and mental wellbeing. The process of meditation involves training the mind to focus and become more aware of the present moment, often through breathing exercises, visualizations, or mindfulness techniques. One of the benefits of meditation is that it can help increase awareness of the flow of Chi within the body.

During meditation, the mind is trained to become increasingly aware of the body's sensations, including the flow of Chi. This increased awareness can help meditators identify areas of blockage or imbalance in the body, which can be addressed through various techniques, such as acupressure. With continued practice, meditators can become more skilled at directing the flow of Chi, which can profoundly affect the body and mind.

However, regular meditation can also help reduce stress, lower blood pressure, and improve overall health and wellbeing. It can help increase feelings of calmness and relaxation, further supporting the body's natural healing processes. In addition, meditation can be a useful tool for those experiencing chronic pain or illness, as it can help reduce symptoms and improve their quality of life.

Studies have shown that regular meditation can increase the production of neurotransmitters, such as serotonin and dopamine, promoting wellbeing and reducing stress and anxiety. Meditation has also been found to reduce inflammation in the body, which is linked to many chronic health conditions, such as heart disease, diabetes, and autoimmune disorders.

In addition to its physical effects, meditation is believed to have spiritual benefits, as well. Many Traditional Chinese Medicine practitioners view Chi cultivation through meditation as a way to connect with the divine and achieve greater levels of consciousness.

Overall, meditation is seen as an important tool in promoting the flow of Chi and achieving balance and harmony in the body and mind. Meditation can be a powerful tool for increasing awareness of the flow of Chi within the body and promoting overall health and wellbeing. With continued practice and dedication, meditators can unlock the full potential of their internal energy and experience profound physical and emotional healing.

Connection Between Chi and the Nervous System

The concept of Chi is closely linked to the nervous system, as it is responsible for regulating the flow of Chi. Essentially, the nervous system transmits signals throughout the body, including signals that control the flow of Chi.

According to Traditional Chinese Medicine, the nervous system and the flow of Chi are connected through a network of channels or meridians that run throughout the body. These channels are believed to be responsible for the distribution of Chi to the body's organs and tissues. When the flow of Chi is disrupted or blocked in these channels, it can lead to various health problems, as previously outlined.

In recent years, there has been increasing scientific interest in the relationship between the nervous system and the flow of Chi. One other form of Eastern medicine that focuses on the connection between Chi and the nervous system is Qigong. It is believed that the practice of Qigong can help balance the nervous system by regulating the sympathetic and parasympathetic branches, which are responsible for the fight or flight response and the rest and digest response, respectively.

Research has shown that the practice of Qigong can have a positive impact on the nervous system. For example, a study published in the *Journal of Alternative and Complementary Medicine* found that Qigong practice was associated with a reduction in stress and anxiety, as well as an increase in heart rate variability, which is a marker of improved autonomic nervous system function. Other studies have found that Qigong can improve cognitive function and reduce symptoms of depression.

Another practice that is believed to influence the flow of Chi and the nervous system includes Tai Chi, which is a form of movement meditation. This practice involves slow, flowing movements that are designed to promote relaxation, balance, and harmony in the body. Studies have shown that Tai Chi can have a range of health benefits, including improvements in balance and flexibility, reductions in stress and anxiety, and improvements in cognitive function.

In addition to these practices, there are a number of other ways in which the flow of Chi and the nervous system can be influenced. For example, certain foods and herbs are believed to have a beneficial effect on the body's Chi, while others may be harmful or disruptive. Massage and other forms of bodywork are also believed to be effective in promoting the flow of Chi and relaxing the nervous system.

Overall, the connection between Chi and the nervous system is a complex and fascinating area of study, with many potential applications in the fields of medicine, psychology, and other health-related disciplines. As research continues to shed light on this relationship, it is likely that we will gain a deeper understanding of the role that Chi plays in maintaining health and wellness, so we can develop new ways of using this knowledge to promote healing and wellbeing.

Connection Between Chi and the Blood

Chi is the vital force that flows through the body and nourishes all the organs and tissues. Similarly, blood is an essential component of the body, responsible for delivering oxygen and nutrients to the cells and removing waste products.

Chi and blood are interconnected and interdependent. Chi is believed to be the driving force behind the movement of blood in the body, whereas blood is said to be the mother of Chi because it provides the nutrients and energy necessary for Chi production.

The relationship between Chi and blood can be illustrated through the concept of meridians, which are linked to the circulatory system, with blood vessels running alongside them. The movement of Chi in the meridians is thought to affect the flow of blood in the corresponding blood vessels.

When Chi is flowing freely through the meridians, it can help regulate the flow of blood and ensure that it reaches all parts of the body. This can help nourish the organs and tissues, supporting overall health and wellbeing. On the other hand, when Chi is blocked or stagnant, it can impede the flow of blood, leading to various health problems.

For example, conditions like high blood pressure, poor circulation, and blood stasis are thought to be caused by an imbalance in the flow of Chi and blood. By addressing the underlying Chi imbalance, the main aim is to improve blood flow and alleviate these conditions.

One way to support the flow of Chi and blood is through techniques like Tai Chi and acupressure. These practices aim to stimulate specific points on the meridians to release blockages and promote the free flow of Chi and blood.

Finally, the free flow of Chi through the meridians has been proven to support the transportation of blood and ensure that it reaches all parts of the body, nourishing the organs and tissues. Addressing any imbalances in Chi can help regulate the flow of blood and improve overall health and wellbeing.

How to Sense Your Chi

Some people are more sensitive to the sensations of Chi, while others may not be as attuned to it. However, everyone has the potential to connect with their Chi and improve its flow.

To better sense your Chi, it is helpful to keep your mind at peace by finding a calm spot. Practices such as meditation or deep breathing exercises can help attain this state. Additionally, regular practice of Qigong, a Chinese exercise system that incorporates movement, breath, and visualization to cultivate and balance Chi, can help improve one's sensitivity to Chi and facilitate its flow.

When the flow of Chi is blocked, it can manifest in various physical symptoms, such as pain, stiffness, or fatigue. By improving one's awareness and sensitivity to Chi, it becomes easier to detect these blockages and take steps to remove them. This can be achieved through practices like acupuncture, which stimulates specific points along the meridians to promote the flow of Chi, and Qigong, which involves various movements and postures designed to facilitate the flow of Chi through the body.

Simple Sign That Your Chi is Blocked

In Traditional Chinese Medicine, the concept of Chi or energy flow is believed to be vital to overall health and wellbeing. When the flow of Chi is blocked or stagnant, it can lead to a variety of physical and mental health issues, as discussed in earlier sections. The reasons for the stagnation of Chi can vary from person to person, but stress and anxiety are some common culprits.

When Chi becomes blocked or stagnated, it slows down the flow of blood, which can lead to various health issues. The symptoms of Chi blockages can vary depending on the location of the blockage. For example, blockages in the kidney organ system, or kidney deficiency, may manifest as memory problems, hair loss, knee pain, back pain, unexplained body aches, and trouble sleeping. Similarly, stagnation in the flow of Chi in the liver can lead to rib pain, upper abdomen fullness, irritability, finger or toenail problems, bitter taste, and muscular pain. It is essential to note that these symptoms of blocked Chi are not exhaustive, and other symptoms may also occur.

Depression, mood swings, inappropriate anger, pain or discomfort in the abdomen, lack of appetite, and fatigue and lethargy are some other symptoms of Chi blockages. Since Chi is the vital energy for the entire body, blockages can have far-reaching effects on overall health and wellbeing.

However, it is possible to unblock or stimulate the flow of Chi through various treatments, such as Qigong and other Traditional Chinese Medicine practices. These practices can help promote relaxation, reduce stress and anxiety, and improve overall energy and vitality, thus restoring the flow of Chi and promoting a healthy body and mind.

Moving and unblocking a blocked Chi

When there are imbalances or blockages in the flow of energy, it can result in pain, exacerbate existing pain, and hinder the body's natural healing processes. To enhance overall wellbeing, it is necessary to restore the free flow of Chi. Traditional Chinese Medicine offers various treatments to unblock and move Chi, thereby improving the body's energy balance.

Acupuncture for addressing Chi stagnation

Acupuncture has been widely recognized as an effective treatment for correcting the flow of Chi and resolving Qi stagnation. Chi stagnation can lead to blockages along the meridian lines, disrupting the smooth flow of both Chi and blood, and causing pain and discomfort in the affected area.

In acupuncture, fine needles are strategically inserted below the skin along the affected meridian lines and areas of blockage to stimulate and move the Chi. The stimulation of these points activates the body's natural healing response, promoting the flow of blood and energy and increasing the body's ability to heal itself.

Clinical studies have shown that acupuncture is an effective modality for treating various pain conditions, including migraines, back and neck pain, carpal tunnel syndrome, arthritis, shoulder pain, fibromyalgia, osteoporosis, pain from injuries, and even cancer pain.

Acupuncture has also been found to be effective in addressing emotional imbalances, such as anxiety and depression, which can also stem from Qi stagnation. Balancing and regulating the flow of Chi can bring a sense of calm and tranquility to the mind and body.

Overall, this practice offers a natural, safe, and effective way to address a wide range of physical and emotional conditions by correcting the flow of Chi and restoring balance to the body's energy system.

Chi blockage herbs

Proper nutrition is vital to support the flow of Chi throughout the body. It is important to avoid processed foods that can prevent nutrient absorption in the gut, which can lead to a deficiency in Chi. Instead, it's best to focus on consuming foods that nourish and sustain the body.

Stews and broths can be particularly beneficial, as can certain herbs that have been used for centuries. For example, if you are experiencing a deficiency in spleen Chi, then herbs like red ginseng, astragalus, jujube dates, licorice, Chinese yam, and pseudostellaria root may be helpful.

To effectively treat liver Chi stagnation, it is not enough to unblock the liver meridian. Other supportive energy systems must also be nourished based on the specific energy needs of the individual. Herbs are often used in combination with others to create formulas that target specific Chi stagnations and support the body's natural healing process.

Some commonly used herbs in the treatment of liver Chi blockages include chai hu (bupleurum), yu jin (turmeric tuber), finger citron fruit (Buddha's Hand), and Xiang fu (cyperus rhizome). These herbs work together to unblock and balance the flow of Chi in the liver, as well as support other energy systems in the body.

By incorporating these herbs into your diet, along with other whole foods, you can support the free flow of Chi throughout your body, leading to improved health and wellbeing.

Treatment by energy professionals

The practice of energy movement arts is a powerful way to move and balance your Chi. Trained healers or practitioners can apply these treatments, while also teaching you how to move your own Chi. Qigong, acupressure, cupping, healing massage, Reiki, and Tai Chi are just a few examples of practices that can be used to strengthen your Chi and unblock its movement.

Qigong is a particularly effective practice for opening the flow of energy in the meridians, enhancing your ability to feel the underlying Chi, and deepening your communication with the life force. This ancient practice uses slow, purposeful techniques that integrate posture, movement, self-massage, breath, and focused intent. With hundreds, if not thousands, of Qigong styles, traditions, and forms practiced around the world through the centuries, this practice remains relevant across the globe. You can find a class near you to learn movements that can help move your Chi.

In addition to energy movement practices, a personalized combination of food, herbal formulas, or acupressure can be used to stimulate the flow of Chi energy in your meridians, restoring balance and health. By working with a knowledgeable practitioner, you can develop a holistic plan that addresses your unique energy needs and helps you achieve optimal wellbeing.

Boosting Your Chi for Optimal Health and Wellness

Sometimes, we drain our Chi without even knowing it; however, they are simple activities that will prepare our body for healing the right way, thus boosting our Chi. Below are some of these activities:

Change your schedule

Excessive social activities and engagements can strain the body and make you feel exhausted. Every day, set aside a minimum of 15 minutes for healthy alone time that fosters rest, introspection, and revitalization. Stay away from places, people, and activities that drain your inner Chi and leave you exhausted. Focus on developing connections with positive people instead.

Declutter

Clutter is a symbol of the heavy, slow-moving Chi energy that keeps us from fulfilling the purpose of our lives. Better, more energetic modifications in the home environment may serve as a springboard for improvements in the financial, professional, and interpersonal spheres. Take control of your clutter, and if you find it impossible, invest money in professional help from a therapist, personal organizer, cleaning service, feng shui expert, or personal organizer.

Breathe deeply

If you breathe shallowly, less energizing oxygen will enter your blood. Put your palm on your stomach while lying on the floor or in bed to practice deep breathing. Keep an eye out for how your hand and stomach both rise as you inhale. Before inhaling again, exhale completely while focusing on your breath.

Fewer desserts

Foods that have been processed, have too much sugar, or include artificial ingredients need to be thrown away. Introduce the following foods instead: seaweed, fermented foods, organic fruits and vegetables, and full-grain foods like oats. Consider tofu, almonds, fish, seeds, and beans for protein instead of red meat and eggs.

How The 24-Hour Chi Cycle Can Help with Diagnosis

Certain principles guide diagnosis and treatment in Traditional Chinese Medicine. Although these principles may seem strange to Westerners, some generalizations can be made to help understand health issues. For example, in terms of the paired organs, let's look at the lungs and large intestines. Often when someone is experiencing bronchitis, asthma, or other respiratory issues, they experience diarrhea. Many people who are nervous, anxious, or fearful—conditions that affect the lungs and breathing—experience lower abdominal cramping. When one has diarrhea, constipation, or a bug in the intestines, they commonly experience breathing issues, especially difficulty taking full breaths. Knowing that the lungs are paired with the large intestines, one can use calming breathing exercises to reduce stomach knots or intestinal pain. When experiencing breathing difficulties, evacuating the bowels offers some immediate relief. One can observe this phenomenon in their own life and that of their clients.

According to Eastern medicine, organ systems have specific times when their energy is at high tide. For example, the lungs are at high tide between the hours of 3 a.m. and 5 a.m. Many people who experience asthma, bronchitis, or other respiratory issues generally find themselves awake and coughing or wheezing between these hours. In TCM, traditionally, the doctor aims to treat the client's ailment when the energy is at its peak for that organ system. This may not be realistic these days, but the client can do things to help themselves during those times with self-directed wellness actions.

The location of the external meridian line (near the skin surface) can also help with diagnosis. For example, those who experience very tight shoulders and necks should consider the possibility that the gallbladder is playing a role. The gallbladder helps support fat digestion. When overworked, gallbladder Qi, or the energy manifested by the gallbladder, may overreact and cause pain and tightness in the gallbladder meridian, which runs along the shoulder and up the back of the neck. Moreover, the gallbladder is paired with the liver, an organ affected by stress. When feeling stressed, our shoulders and neck tend to tense up.

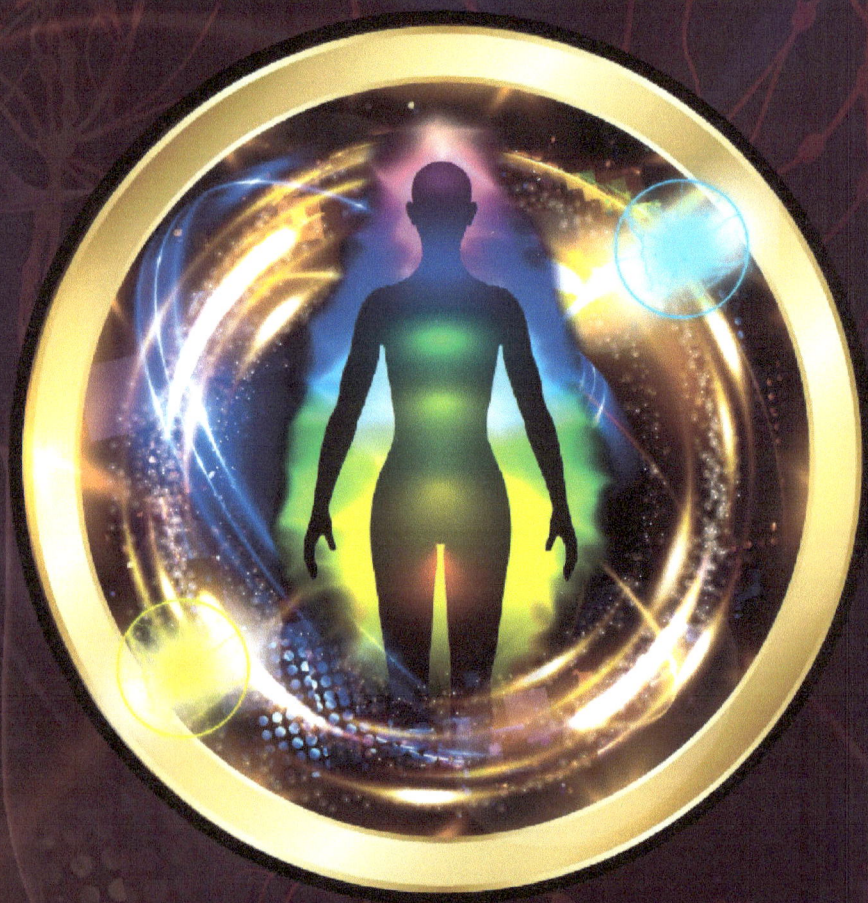

02

SCIENTIFIC EVIDENCE OF CHI

For centuries, the concept of Chi has been a central tenet of Traditional Chinese Medicine and other Eastern healing practices. Chi, also known as Qi or Ki, is often described as a vital energy or life force that flows through the body and animates all living things. Despite its long-standing presence in Eastern cultures, the existence and properties of Chi have been met with skepticism and scrutiny in Western medicine and science.

However, recent advances in technology and research have provided compelling evidence to support the existence of Chi and its importance in maintaining health and wellness. This section of the book will explore the scientific evidence of Chi and its potential applications in modern medicine and healing practices. We will examine the research findings and scientific explanations behind the concept of Chi and its effects on the body, mind, and spirit.

Confirmation of the Existence of Chi

The concept that the body possesses a system of channels through which energy flows is pervasive throughout ancient thought. When reinforced by meditation or other similar techniques, this energy has a positive impact on health and has the capacity to exert power—it may be utilized to deliver strikes in martial arts, in some cases.

It was known as Mana in Polynesia, Ka in Egypt, Ki in Japan, Ruach in Jewish mysticism, Prana in India, Chi or Qi in China, and, more recently, Élan Vital or Subtle Energy in the West.

Prana, Chi, Subtle Energy, and—in the more tongue-twisting contemporary scientific jargon, bioelectromagnetism—are just a few of the numerous names for this enigmatic but potent energy in the human body.

The human body employs electricity; for instance, our senses use electrical currents to transmit data to the brain. Whenever an electric charge is moving, a magnetic field is produced. In other words, bioelectromagnetism is the electromagnetic field produced by currents flowing through our bodies. Some scientists and Chi practitioners claim that this could be Chi.

Christopher Dow, in one of his books, *The Wellspring: An Inquiry Into the Nature of Chi,* said that the bioelectromagnetism that envelops nerve pathways is Chi. Therefore, the Chi does not flow down the nerve by itself but instead creates an invisible zone that may be somewhat controlled around the electrical flow.

This basically means that he has learned much of what science says about electromagnetic energy flow through the body. Also, Dow has noticed some significant parallels between how the neurological system functions and what has long been preached about Chi channels. For instance, the "tantien" or "dantian" in the lower abdomen is a vital location for Chi in the body. This relates to the strong nerve center in the gut called the Enteric Plexus.

The Enteric Plexus, also known as the intrinsic nervous system of the gut, plays a crucial role in the regulation of the gastrointestinal system. It consists of a complex network of nerves that are located in the walls of the digestive tract, from the esophagus to the anus. These nerves control various functions, such as peristalsis, secretion, blood flow, and nutrient absorption.

One of the important roles of the Enteric Plexus is its interaction with the lymphatic system. The lymphatic system is a network of vessels and organs that helps in the maintenance of fluid balance and immune function. The lymphatic vessels in the digestive tract absorb the fats and lipid-soluble vitamins that are not absorbed by the blood vessels.

The Enteric Plexus helps in the regulation of the lymphatic system by controlling the contractions of the lymphatic vessels. The enteric nervous system secretes several neurotransmitters that control the tone and contraction of the smooth muscles in the wall of the lymphatic vessels. The contraction of these muscles helps move the lymphatic fluid toward the lymph nodes, where it is filtered and purified before returning to the bloodstream.

Moreover, the Enteric Plexus also interacts with the immune cells that are present in the gut-associated lymphoid tissue (GALT). The GALT is a vital component of the immune system that protects the body against harmful microorganisms and pathogens. The enteric plexus regulates the migration of immune cells towards the GALT, while also influencing the secretion of cytokines and other immune mediators that help in the coordination of the immune response.

Overall, the Enteric Plexus plays a critical role in the regulation of the lymphatic system by controlling the contraction of the lymphatic vessels and interacting with the immune cells present in the gut-associated lymphoid tissue. The proper functioning of the Enteric Plexus is essential for the maintenance of digestive and immune health. This is why, as a Chi component, it is very important. However, to further buttress the proof of the existence of Chi, below are some other backings:

Science and wisdom: Same truth but different approaches

Chris Dow once highlighted that "both science and the esoteric traditions seek the truth; they simply go at it in different ways, and that is because the Esoteric traditions don't just appear out of nowhere." According to him, they include specific methodologies that are taught from instructor to student, much as in science.

Science wants to be able to declare, "This is how it is," and prove it unequivocally to all of us. This is one of the distinctions. Esoteric traditions, on the other hand, have a tendency to remain isolated. You may demonstrate the energy to yourself and assist others in discovering it, but you can't write a paper and expect everyone to grasp it since, according to esoteric traditions, you must discover it for yourself.

He knows this energy exists because he has experienced it profoundly in his body as a student of Chi. That inspired him to research the subject scientifically.

Dow doubts that Western science will ever be able to identify Chi. He stated, "It could be that the only instrument that can measure this is the human body."

Body bioenergy force and extreme sensitive pendulum swing

Dr. John Norman Hansen, a biochemist at the University of Maryland, discovered that the human body has a bioenergy force around it that can move a torsion pendulum, a particularly sensitive pendulum.

In his 2013 study titled, "Use of a Torsion Pendulum Balance to Detect and Characterize What May Be a Human Bioenergy Field," he wrote, "After conducting control experiments to rule out effects of air currents and other artifacts, it is concluded that the effects are exerted by some kind of force field that is generated by the subject seated under the pendulum."

Nothing in contemporary mainstream science, he pointed out, explains how the pendulum swings. The way Chi is traditionally understood, it not only flows through the body's internal pathways but also creates a field all around it.

Heart energy can influence others

Researchers from the HeartMath Institute and Stanford University Professor Emeritus Dr. William Tiller have shown that the electromagnetic field of the heart may "become more coherent as the individual shifts to a sincerely loving or caring state." An ECG, a test that tracks the electrical activity of the heart, was used to quantify this field.

Additionally, these researchers have shown that when two people are in close proximity or contact, the electromagnetic field of one person's heart impacts the energy in the other person's body.

Again, this is consistent with conventional views of Chi, which maintain that both one's own Chi and the Chi of others are influenced by one's mental state.

Phantom limb phenomenon: Does intangible energy truly exist in the body?

People who have lost a limb often still feel it, sometimes to the point of experiencing excruciating agony. Theoretically, phantom limbs might be energetic forms that persist, according to Dr. Eric Leskowitz, a consultant psychiatrist to the Spaulding Rehabilitation Hospital in Boston's pain management program and an expert in subtle energy.

He uses anecdotal data gathered via Kirlian photography in his study titled, "Phantom Limb Pain: Subtle Energy Perspectives." This style of photography depicts colorful rings of light around its objects, which are sometimes called "auras."

However, other people are suspicious of the "aura" explanation, contending that this light effect is actually caused by heat or moisture. To explain this experimental finding, a non-local process or field must be invoked, even if the corona is an artifact of heat or moisture rather than a subtle energy event.

He pointed out that phantom limbs could be related to the contentious "phantom leaf" phenomena. In Kirlian images, a ripped leaf sometimes seems to have a full energy pattern, undisturbed by the amputation.

Near invisible network channels in the body

According to Leskowitz, the energetic grid that maintains the leaf tip is still there even after its physical counterpart is taken away.

The phantom leaf phenomenon was replicated in research that John Hubacher of Pantheon Research Inc. published in the *Journal of Alternative and Complementary Medicine* in 2015. In his writing, he said that "a normally undetected phantom structure, possibly evidence of the biological field, can persist in the area of an amputated leaf section, and corona discharge can occur from this invisible structure."

According to some researchers, the body possesses an ultra-microscopic network of Chi-channel-corresponding channels.

More studies have been conducted in recent years on a hypothesized "primo-vascular system."

The body has a network of channels that are so tiny they are essentially invisible. "Even with our microscope, the vessels are clear, so you cannot see them until you touch them;

nonetheless, when touched, they take on a yellowish hue. The node is barely one millimeter across, and high-resolution light microscopy is the only way to observe the node's intricate structure," according to a news release from Vitaly Vodyanoy of Auburn University. The College of Veterinary Medicine's anatomy and physiology professor, Vodyanoy, has investigated this structure in rats.

According to Vodyanoy, "We are pushing the limits of accepted or recognized anatomy and physiology." The primo-vascular system is not often studied since it contradicts accepted scientific theories.

The primo-vascular system is described as follows by an international team of researchers, some of whom are from Seoul National University: "Some scientists may say it is an illusion; others say it is a 'new' anatomical system; still others are convinced that these infinitesimal channels may act like optical fiber cables and transmit DNA related information continuously throughout the body using biophotons."

We cannot see the millions of transistors on a CPU (central processing unit), but they are a component of a system that was created by humans that we use every day. Similar to this, a lot of biological systems are really quite little. To see some of their structures, we require electronic microscopes; otherwise, we wouldn't be aware that they exist. These scientists investigate the evidence that the primo-vascular system and acupuncture meridians are related.

Chi has long been believed to have a direct impact on how healthy one's physique is. According to a statement from the Institute of Noetic Sciences, studies of the Chi exercise known as Qigong have shown favorable health benefits in areas including depression, pain management, asthma, cancer, and blood pressure.

Studies on meditation, which is said to improve Chi, have shown that those who practice it may generate gamma and infrasonic waves above normal levels.

The body possesses energy channels and a field that affects a person's health and the environment around them, which may be supported by science's ongoing research of the body's energy, its flow, and its consequences.

In recent years, there have been numerous scientific studies that support the existence of Chi in the body. One area of research that has gained a lot of attention is bioelectricity. Bioelectricity refers to the electrical signals that are generated by living organisms. It is now widely accepted that the body has a complex system of electrical currents that help regulate various physiological processes. This system is thought to be closely connected to the body's Chi energy system.

Similarly, several studies have been conducted to explore the mechanisms behind acupuncture and the role of Chi in this practice. For instance, a study published in the *Journal of Alternative and Complementary Medicine* in 2010 found that acupuncture can modulate the activity of the autonomic nervous system, which is responsible for regulating various bodily functions, including blood pressure and heart rate. Another study published in the *Journal of Acupuncture and Meridian Studies* in 2013 showed that acupuncture can stimulate the release of endorphins and other neurotransmitters, which can help to reduce pain and improve mood.

In addition to these findings, researchers have also used modern imaging techniques, such as functional magnetic resonance imaging (fMRI) and positron emission tomography (PET), to investigate the effects of acupuncture on the brain. One study, published in *Nature Neuroscience* in 2002, used fMRI to show that acupuncture can activate specific regions of the brain involved in pain perception and processing.

In the same light, Qigong research has also demonstrated the existence of Chi energy in the body. In a study published in the *Journal of Alternative and Complementary Medicine* in 2004, researchers found that Qigong can increase the electrical conductivity of the skin, which is thought to be related to the flow of Chi energy in the body.

Qigong has gained attention in recent years as a practice that promotes physical and mental health. There have been several studies that support the existence of Chi and the positive effects of Qigong on the body. Qigong practice also improves immune function in breast cancer clients undergoing radiotherapy. The study found that Qigong practice resulted in significant increases in levels of white blood cells and natural killer cells, which play a crucial role in immune function.

Another study published in the *Journal of Psychiatric Research* in 2016 investigated the effects of Qigong on depression and anxiety in clients with chronic obstructive pulmonary disease (COPD). The study found that Qigong practice significantly improved depression and anxiety symptoms in the participants, suggesting that the practice may have a positive effect on mental health.

In addition to these studies, there have been numerous other investigations into the effects of Qigong on various health conditions, such as chronic pain, hypertension, and Parkinson's disease. While the exact mechanisms behind Qigong are still being explored, it is believed that the practice helps balance and regulate the flow of Chi energy in the body, promoting overall health and wellbeing.

Ultimately, the scientific evidence for the existence of Chi in the body is growing, and many researchers believe that further studies in this area could have important implications for the treatment of various health conditions. While there is still much to learn about the nature of Chi energy and its role in the body, the evidence suggests that this ancient concept may have a place in modern medicine.

How these studies have led to a better understanding of the physiological mechanisms of Chi in the body

The research on bioelectricity has provided valuable insights into the physiological mechanisms of Chi in the body. Bioelectricity studies have revealed that the body's cells generate electrical fields that can be modulated by external fields. This suggests that the flow of Chi in the body may be linked to the generation and modulation of electrical fields within the body's cells.

For example, studies have shown that acupuncture can cause changes in neurotransmitters, hormones, and immune system activity, all of which are important for the regulation of various bodily functions. These findings suggest that it may work by stimulating specific physiological pathways in the body that are linked to the flow of Chi.

Similarly, Qigong research has revealed that this practice can influence the autonomic nervous system, the endocrine system, and the immune system. These systems are all closely interconnected and are involved in regulating various physiological processes, such as heart rate, hormone production, and immune function. By influencing these systems, Qigong may promote the smooth flow of Chi in the body and improve overall health and wellbeing.

Overall, the research on bioelectricity has contributed to a better understanding of the physiological mechanisms of Chi in the body. These studies suggest that the flow of Chi may be linked to the modulation of electrical fields within the body's cells and the stimulation of specific physiological pathways that are involved in regulating bodily functions. By harnessing the power of Chi, individuals may be able to promote optimal health and wellbeing.

These studies have helped bridge the gap between Traditional Chinese Medicine and Western medicine by providing scientific evidence for the existence of Chi and its effects on the body. They have also led to the development of new therapies and treatments that incorporate principles of Traditional Chinese Medicine, such as Qigong, into mainstream medical practice. Overall, the scientific research on Chi has opened up new avenues for understanding and treating a wide range of health conditions and has helped validate the importance of Traditional Chinese Medicine in promoting health and wellbeing.

How healthcare practitioners Integrate Chi-based therapies into their practice, including Tai Chi and Qigong

In recent years, there has been an increasing interest among healthcare practitioners in incorporating Chi-based therapies into their practice. Tai Chi and Qigong are among the most commonly used therapies.

Tai Chi

Tai Chi is a traditional Chinese martial art that has gained popularity worldwide as a form of exercise and meditation. It involves a series of slow, flowing movements that are designed to improve flexibility, balance, and strength, while also promoting relaxation and stress reduction. Tai Chi is often referred to as "moving meditation" because it involves both physical and mental focus.

Studies have shown that Tai Chi can be beneficial for a range of health conditions, including arthritis, heart disease, and depression. One study found that Tai Chi can help reduce the risk of falls in older adults, while another study found that it can improve sleep quality in people with chronic insomnia. Tai Chi has also been shown to be effective in reducing anxiety and depression in cancer patients.

Qigong

Qigong is another gentle exercise that is similar to Tai Chi but is focused more specifically on the cultivation and regulation of Chi energy. Qigong exercises involve slow, repetitive movements, deep breathing, and meditation, and are designed to improve overall health and wellbeing by balancing and enhancing the flow of Chi in the body.

Research has shown that Qigong can be effective in reducing stress and anxiety, improving balance and coordination, and boosting immune function. One study found that Qigong was effective in reducing the symptoms of fibromyalgia, while another study found that it can help improve cognitive function in older adults.

Some healthcare practitioners have also started to incorporate mindfulness-based practices, such as meditation and deep breathing exercises, into their practice to help clients reduce stress and improve overall wellbeing. These practices have been shown to be effective in reducing anxiety, improving sleep quality, and enhancing immune function.

As more research is conducted on the physiological mechanisms of Chi-based therapies, healthcare practitioners are gaining a better understanding of how these practices can be used to promote health and wellbeing. Many healthcare institutions have also started to offer Chi-based therapies as part of their integrative medicine programs, allowing clients to benefit from a range of complementary approaches to healthcare.

Astrology/Divination

These allow us to clear the mind of worrying and regret.

Remember: You cannot change the past and trying to will only interfere with the flow of energy of moving forward.

Incorporating Chi-based therapies into medical practice, like astrology and divination, can be used as a means of helping clients clear their minds and focus on moving forward.

Astrology and divination are often used as tools for self-reflection and introspection. By analyzing patterns and symbols, clients may be able to gain insight into their own thought patterns and emotional responses. This can be especially helpful for clients who are struggling with anxiety, depression, or other mental health issues.

Practitioners who integrate astrology and divination into their practice can use these metaphysical tools in different ways. For example, they may use astrology to help clients understand their astrological chart and how it may be influencing their life. They may use tarot cards or other divination tools to help clients gain insight into their current situation or help them make decisions about the future.

That being said, it is important to note that while astrology and divination can be helpful tools for self-reflection and introspection, they are not a substitute for traditional medical care.

Feng shui

Feng shui is an ancient Chinese practice that involves arranging the environment to promote harmony and balance in the flow of energy or Chi. Healthcare practitioners may integrate feng shui principles into their practice to help their clients achieve optimal health and wellness.

Creating a home or work environment that supports the flow of energy can help reduce stress, improve creativity, and enhance overall wellbeing. For instance, placing plants or natural elements in the workplace can help improve air quality and promote a sense of calmness. Using color and lighting to create a peaceful atmosphere can also be beneficial for mental and emotional health.

Moreover, incorporating feng shui principles can help healthcare practitioners better understand their clients' needs and how to create a healing environment that supports their physical, emotional, and spiritual health. By understanding how the energy flows in a particular space, practitioners can make adjustments to promote healing and reduce stress.

Improving Client Results and Supporting Overall Health

Many traditional healing practices, such as acupuncture and Qigong, have gained popularity in recent years as complementary and alternative therapies for a variety of health conditions. These practices are rooted in the concept of a subtle energy force that flows through the body, and the manipulation of this energy is believed to promote health and healing. The nearly invisible network channels, or meridians, through which this energy flows can be stimulated through acupuncture and Qigong to promote the smooth flow of this energy and improve overall wellness. Additionally, these therapies have been shown to have a positive impact on the body's bioenergy force and heart energy, both of which are important for maintaining good health. Furthermore, these practices can be beneficial in addressing phantom limb pain, a phenomenon that is believed to be related to disruptions in the body's bioenergy force. Overall, these therapies have the potential to improve client outcomes and support overall health by promoting the body's natural healing mechanisms and rebalancing its energy systems.

In addition to pain relief, acupuncture can also promote relaxation and reduce stress and anxiety. This is because the therapy has been shown to activate the parasympathetic nervous system, which is responsible for the body's relaxation response. Acupuncture can also help balance the body's hormones and neurotransmitters, which can improve mood and overall mental health.

Qigong

Qigong is a low-impact form of exercise that involves a series of slow, gentle movements, deep breathing, and meditation. It is considered a mind-body practice that can help promote a sense of calm and relaxation, while also improving physical health. Studies have shown that regular Qigong practice can have a positive impact on a range of health issues, including hypertension, diabetes, and chronic pain. Additionally, the gentle movements involved in Qigong can help improve balance and flexibility, making it a particularly useful form of exercise for older adults or those with limited mobility, as previously mentioned. Overall, Qigong can be a valuable addition to a wellness routine and may help to improve overall physical and mental health.

Near invisible network channels, also known as meridians or energy pathways

In Traditional Chinese Medicine, the concept of meridians or energy pathways has been recognized for thousands of years. These pathways are believed to be a network of channels that run throughout the body, carrying the body's vital energy or life force, known as Chi. The meridians are thought to connect the body's organs, muscles, and tissues, creating a complex network that is responsible for the flow of Chi throughout the body.

The manipulation of these channels is the foundation of many traditional Chinese medical practices, including acupuncture and Qigong. Acupuncture involves the insertion of thin needles into specific points along the meridians to stimulate the flow of Chi and promote healing. Qigong, on the other hand, involves gentle exercises and movements that help balance the flow of Chi throughout the body, promoting overall health and wellbeing.

Recent research has provided some evidence to support the existence of meridians and the role they play in the body. For example, a study published in the *Journal of Acupuncture and Meridian Studies* found that the stimulation of acupuncture points along specific meridians resulted in changes in brain activity, suggesting a direct link between the meridians and the central nervous system.

Other studies have found that the manipulation of the meridians through practices such as acupuncture and Qigong can have a range of health benefits. For example, a study published in the *Journal of Alternative and Complementary Medicine* found that acupuncture was effective in reducing pain and improving function in clients with knee osteoarthritis. Another study published in the *Journal of Gerontology* found that Qigong was effective in reducing falls and improving balance in older adults.

Overall, the concept of meridians and the manipulation of energy pathways is an important component of Traditional Chinese Medicine, and recent research has provided some evidence to support their existence and the role they play in the body. By promoting the smooth flow of Chi through these pathways, practices such as acupuncture and Qigong can help improve overall health and wellbeing.

The phantom limb phenomenon

As briefly discussed earlier, this phenomenon occurs when an individual experiences sensations or pain in a limb that has been amputated and is thought to be related to disruptions in the body's bioenergy force.

Research suggests that acupuncture and Qigong can be effective in reducing phantom limb pain. In a study published in the *Journal of Rehabilitation Medicine,* researchers found that acupuncture was effective in reducing pain and improving the quality of life in clients with phantom limb pain. Similarly, a study published in *Pain Medicine* found that Qigong was effective in reducing phantom limb pain and improving overall wellbeing in amputee clients. These therapies are believed to work by promoting the flow of Chi and restoring balance to the body's bioenergy force, which can help alleviate the symptoms of phantom limb pain.

In addition to acupuncture and Qigong, there are other therapies that have been shown to be effective in reducing the symptoms of phantom limb pain. One such therapy is mirror therapy, which involves using a mirror to create the illusion that the amputated limb is still present. The client then performs exercises with the intact limb while watching the reflection in the mirror, which can help alleviate phantom limb pain. Another therapy is transcutaneous electrical nerve stimulation (TENS), which involves the use of electrical stimulation to disrupt pain signals and promote the release of endorphins, the body's natural painkillers. These therapies, in combination with acupuncture and Qigong, can provide a holistic approach to managing phantom limb pain and improving the overall quality of life for individuals with amputations.

Heart energy

Research has demonstrated that the heart's electromagnetic field is not only the strongest electromagnetic field generated by the body but also has a broader reach than previously thought. The heart's electromagnetic field can influence other people's emotional states and physiological processes. Studies have also shown that the heart's electromagnetic field can change with emotional states, such as anxiety or relaxation. A healthy heart energy field, characterized by coherence in the heart rate variability, has been associated with lower levels of stress, improved immune system function, and lower risk of heart disease and other health problems.

Practices such as meditation and deep breathing exercises have been shown to help promote a healthy heart energy field. For example, research has found that mindfulness meditation can lead to increased coherence in heart rate variability and improved emotional regulation. Similarly, practices such as deep breathing exercises, particularly those that involve longer exhales than inhales, have been shown to improve heart rate variability and reduce stress levels. These practices can be used to support overall health and wellbeing, particularly in the areas of stress management and cardiovascular health.

The body's bioenergy force

In addition to stress, poor nutrition, and environmental toxins, other factors can also disrupt the body's bioenergy force, including illness, injury, and emotional trauma. When this force is disrupted, it can lead to imbalances in the body's physiological processes, resulting in a range of symptoms and conditions.

Therapies such as acupuncture, acupressure, and Qigong are believed to work by restoring balance to the body's bioenergy force, which can, in turn, improve overall health and wellbeing. By stimulating specific points along the body's meridians or energy pathways, acupuncture can help regulate the flow of Chi and promote healing. Similarly, Qigong exercises can help increase the body's energy flow and promote relaxation and balance.

Studies have shown that these therapies can be effective in reducing pain, improving immune function, and enhancing overall wellbeing. Improving the body's bioenergy force through acupuncture and Qigong can help promote better sleep, reduce stress and anxiety, and support emotional health. Overall, these therapies offer a holistic approach to healthcare, addressing not just physical symptoms but also emotional and mental aspects of health.

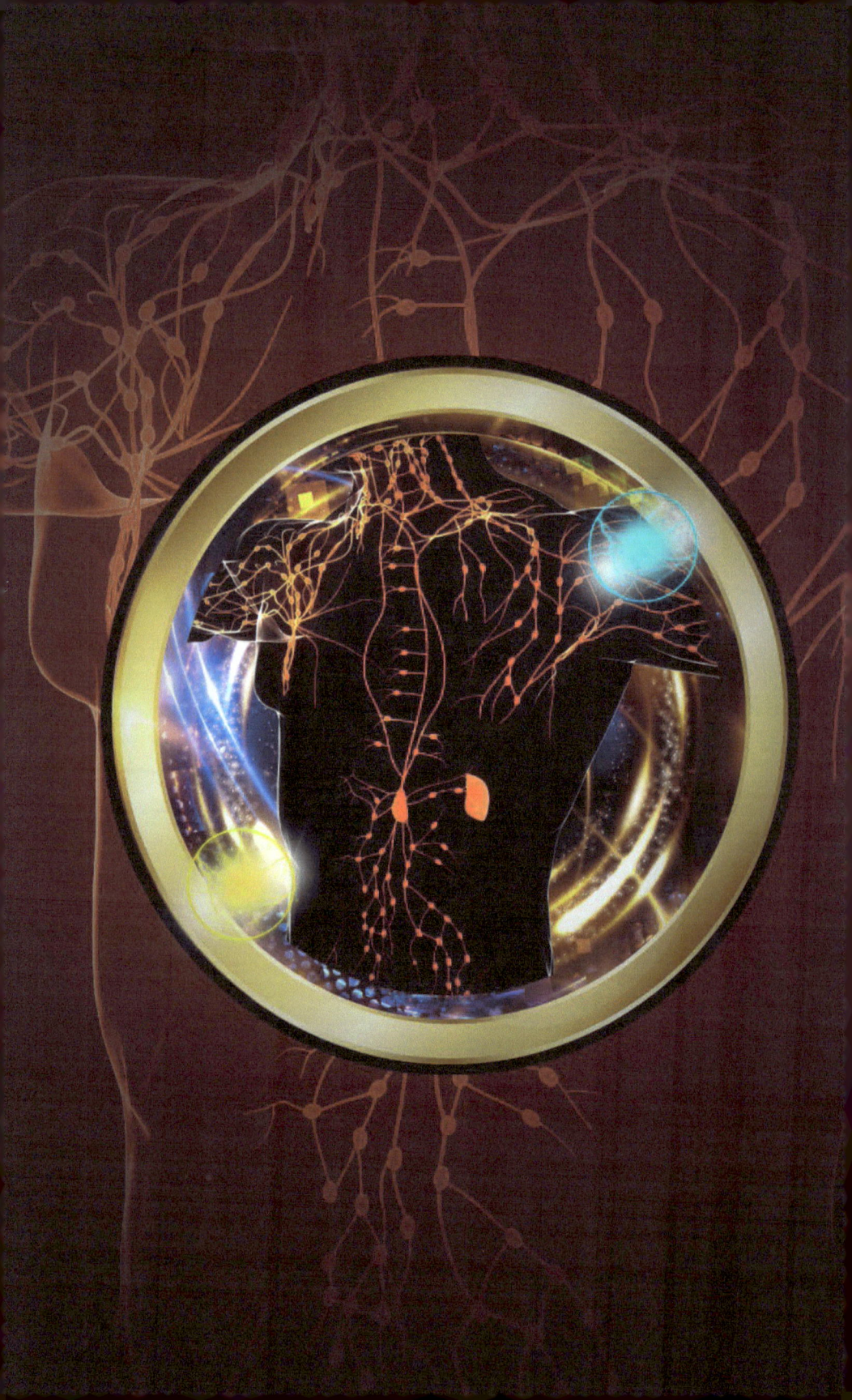

03

UNDERSTANDING THE LYMPHATIC SYSTEM

The lymphatic system is a critical part of the body's immune system, and its functions are crucial for maintaining a healthy body. However, it is often overshadowed by the more popular circulatory system, which is responsible for the transportation of blood throughout the body. In this chapter, we will dive deep into the physiology of the lymphatic system, how it is connected to other systems in the body, and its essential role in the immune system.

Furthermore, we will explore the importance of lymphatic treatment, which can help improve the function of the lymphatic system, reduce inflammation, and improve overall health. We will also discuss blockages in the lymphatic system and how they can affect the body, leading to various health problems.

It is crucial to understand that the lymphatic system plays a critical role in the whole mind, body, brain, soul, and spirit, and that it is not associated with any specific religion. So, whether you are a health enthusiast, a medical professional, or someone who is curious about the workings of the human body, this chapter will provide you with valuable insights into the importance of the lymphatic system and how it can impact your health and wellbeing.

The Physiology of the Lymphatic System

The lymphatic system is an essential component of the body's immune system. It is responsible for maintaining fluid balance, filtering out harmful substances, and protecting the body against infections and diseases. The lymphatic system consists of a network of lymphatic vessels, lymph nodes, and lymphatic organs, including the spleen, thymus, and tonsils.

Lymphatic vessels are similar in structure to veins, but they carry a clear, colorless fluid called lymph. Lymph is a mixture of water, proteins, and waste products, and it is formed from the fluid that leaks out of blood vessels and into the surrounding tissues. Lymphatic vessels collect this fluid and transport it through the lymphatic system, where it is filtered and cleansed before being returned to the bloodstream.

Lymph nodes are small, bean-shaped structures that are found throughout the body but are concentrated in certain areas, such as the neck, armpits, and groin. Lymph nodes act as filters, removing foreign particles, such as bacteria, viruses, and cancer cells, from the lymph before it is returned to the bloodstream. When the body is fighting an infection or disease, lymph nodes may become swollen and tender as the immune system produces more lymphocytes to attack the invading organisms.

The spleen is the largest lymphatic organ in the body, and it is responsible for filtering blood and removing old or damaged red blood cells. The thymus is a gland located in the chest, which plays a critical role in the development of T-cells, a type of white blood cell that is important in fighting infections.

The tonsils are another lymphatic organ that helps protect the body against infections. They are located in the back of the throat and are part of the body's first line of defense against bacteria and viruses that enter through the mouth and nose.

The lymphatic system is also connected to other systems in the body, including the cardiovascular system and the digestive system. Lymphatic vessels are closely associated with blood vessels, and they work together to maintain fluid balance in the body. The lymphatic system also plays a role in the absorption of fats and fat-soluble vitamins from the digestive tract.

Overall, we can say that the lymphatic system is a vital part of the body's immune system. It helps protect the body against infections and diseases, maintains fluid balance, and works in conjunction with other systems in the body to maintain overall health and wellness.

Development of Cancer and the Lymphatic System

Our defense against the development of cancer depends on the lymphatic system. Swollen lymph nodes may be a symptom that a malignant tumor is present; however, this isn't always the case. This is because when cancer cells escape from a tumor, they might get stuck within a neighboring lymph node. When a patient is tested for cancer, or an investigation is conducted to determine whether an existing malignancy has spread, the first step is to check the lymph nodes for inflammation and other abnormalities.

The production of lymphocytes, a few of which produce antibodies—proteins that kill microorganisms and prevent the spread of illnesses or altered cells—is a crucial function of the immune system. In certain cases, this procedure is too slow to combat free radical damage and halt the progression of cancer. Alternately, dysfunctional and mutated cells may begin to multiply and spread quickly.

Lymph node cancer, often known as lymphoma, may either originate there or spread from another location. Through the blood or lymph fluid, cancer cells that have detached from a tumor can move to other parts of the body, where they can reach other organs and continue to grow.

The body usually manages this process and can eliminate small amounts of mutated cells or cancerous cells that have escaped before they spread, but it only takes a few mutated cancerous cells to travel to another part of the body before they can form new tumors (a process known as metastasis). If lymph nodes enlarge, this can become painful and obvious very quickly (sometimes they are big and tender enough to feel with your fingers by pushing on the skin).

The stage of a person's cancer and the treatment options depend on whether the disease has spread to the lymph nodes. If a lymph node gets contaminated with cancer cells, a surgeon may remove it (this is known as a biopsy), or if it is too late because the disease has spread, additional therapies like chemotherapy or radiation may be required. One concern with removing lymph nodes to eliminate cancer cells is that this prevents the body from maintaining fluid balance and eliminating tissue waste, which may result in tissue swelling and hurting, a condition known as lymphedema.

The acronym "TNM system" (tumor, metastasis, and [lymph] nodes) is used by many clinicians to categorize the various stages of cancer. A score of 0 indicates that there is no lymph node cancer; a number between 1-3 indicates that the cancer is present but not yet severe; and a value of 3-4 indicates that the cancer is in the "late-stage" range.

Lymphatic System, Inner Energy, and Connectivity with Other Systems

The lymphatic system is closely interconnected with several other systems in the body, including the circulatory system, immune system, and the Chi energy system.

The circulatory system and the lymphatic system work together to maintain fluid balance in the body. Blood carries oxygen and nutrients to the cells, and the lymphatic system removes excess fluid and waste products from the tissues. The lymphatic vessels also help return the excess fluid to the bloodstream, which is then circulated back to the heart.

The immune system and the lymphatic system are also closely intertwined. The lymph nodes act as filters, trapping and removing harmful bacteria, viruses, and other foreign substances from the body. The lymphatic system transports these substances to the lymph nodes, where they are destroyed by white blood cells. The lymphatic system also plays a role in the production of white blood cells, which are critical for fighting infections and diseases.

Traditional Chinese Medicine views the lymphatic system as an integral part of the body's energy system. The lymphatic vessels are believed to be pathways for the flow of Chi throughout the body, and when this flow is disrupted, it can lead to blockages in the lymphatic system and impaired immune function. Conversely, when the flow of Chi is balanced and harmonious, the lymphatic system can function optimally, promoting health and wellbeing.

One of the key ways that the lymphatic system is connected to other systems in the body is through its relationship with the circulatory system. The lymphatic vessels work in tandem with the blood vessels to transport fluids and nutrients throughout the body. The lymphatic vessels absorb excess fluid, waste products, and debris from the body's tissues and transport them to the lymph nodes for filtration and removal. This process helps maintain a healthy balance of fluids and nutrients in the body.

The lymphatic system also plays a vital role in the immune system, helping to identify and remove foreign invaders, such as bacteria and viruses. The lymph nodes are the sites where immune cells are produced and activated, and they play a key role in fighting infections and other diseases.

In Traditional Chinese Medicine, blockages in the lymphatic system are believed to result from imbalances in the body's energy system. These imbalances can be caused by factors such as stress, poor diet, lack of exercise, and environmental toxins. Practices like any type of lymphatic treatment are used to help balance the flow of Chi and promote lymphatic health.

Most types of lymphatic treatment involve the use of gentle massage techniques to stimulate the flow of lymphatic fluid and remove blockages. The therapist uses light, rhythmic strokes to massage the lymphatic vessels and encourage the flow of lymphatic fluid toward the lymph nodes. This helps reduce swelling, improve immune function, and promote overall wellbeing.

In conclusion, the lymphatic system is an essential part of the body's overall function, closely interconnected with the circulatory and immune systems, as well as the Chi energy system in Traditional Chinese Medicine. Understanding the relationship between these systems and how they work together can help to promote optimal health and wellbeing.

Importance of Chi to the Lymphatic System

In Traditional Chinese Medicine, the flow of Chi energy is believed to be closely connected to the lymphatic system. When the flow of Chi is disrupted, it can lead to blockages in the lymphatic system and impaired immune function. On the other hand, when the flow of Chi is balanced and harmonious, the lymphatic system can function optimally, promoting health and wellbeing.

Therefore, harnessing the power of Chi can be beneficial for the lymphatic system. This can be achieved through various practices, such as meditation, deep breathing exercises, sound therapy, walking in nature, and Qigong, to name a few.

Meditation and deep breathing exercises have been practiced for centuries and are known to provide numerous health benefits. In the context of lymphatic treatment, these practices can be particularly effective in promoting the flow of lymph and reducing blockages. Meditation involves focusing the mind on a particular object or thought, often through guided imagery or mindfulness techniques. Through meditation, the body can enter a state of deep relaxation, which can help reduce stress and anxiety levels. This, in turn, can have a positive effect on the lymphatic system, as stress and tension can cause blockages and impair the flow of lymphatic fluid. Deep breathing exercises, such as diaphragmatic breathing or pranayama, involve breathing deeply and slowly from the abdomen. This type of breathing can improve the flow of oxygen throughout the body and promote relaxation, which can, in turn, improve lymphatic healing. Deep breathing exercises can also help stimulate the lymphatic system by creating a gentle pressure that moves the lymphatic fluid. This can help improve overall health and wellbeing, reduce the risk of disease, and enhance the effectiveness of lymphatic recovery therapies.

In addition to these practices, maintaining a healthy diet and lifestyle can also help promote the flow of Chi. Eating a diet rich in fruits, vegetables, and whole grains can provide the body with essential nutrients and antioxidants that help support lymphatic function. Regular exercise, getting enough rest, and staying hydrated are all important for overall wellness and lymphatic health.

In summary, harnessing the power of Chi through practices such as meditation, deep breathing exercises, and maintaining a healthy lifestyle can help improve lymphatic flow and overall wellness.

Blockages in the Lymphatic System and How They Affect the Body

As discussed, the lymphatic system plays a critical role in maintaining a healthy immune system, and blockages in the system can have negative impacts on overall health and wellbeing. Blockages in the lymphatic system can be caused by a variety of factors, including injury, surgery, infections, inflammation, and even stress.

These blockages in the lymphatic system can lead to a range of health problems. When lymphatic vessels become blocked or damaged, lymphatic fluid can accumulate and cause swelling or edema in the affected area. This can occur in any part of the body but is most commonly seen in the arms, legs, and feet.

When the lymphatic system becomes blocked, it can result in a buildup of lymphatic fluid, which can cause swelling, pain, and discomfort. In severe cases, blockages can lead to a condition known as lymphedema, which is characterized by chronic swelling in a specific area of the body, often the limbs.

Blockages in the lymphatic system can also have broader impacts on the body's immune function. The lymphatic system is responsible for filtering and removing waste products and toxins from the body, and when the system is blocked, these substances can accumulate, leading to further health complications.

Fortunately, there are a variety of therapies that can help unblock the lymphatic system and promote healthy lymphatic flow.

That being said, people with lymphatic blocks may not recover quickly because the lymphatic system is closely connected to the immune system. When the lymphatic system is blocked, the immune system's ability to fight off infections and diseases is compromised. This makes it harder for the body to recover from illnesses or injuries, further slowing down the recovery process.

It is important to address blockages in the lymphatic system as early as possible to prevent further complications and promote overall health and wellness. With the right therapies and techniques, it is possible to restore healthy lymphatic flow and support a strong and resilient immune system.

Why Lymph-Chi Treatment is Essential for Blockage Removal

As a holistic health approach to overall wellness, Lymph-Chi aims to not only remove physical lymphatic blockages in the physical body, but also in the metaphysical body. The approach emphasizes the importance of the interconnectivity of the body's systems and organs, including the meridians, in achieving optimal health.

The treatment involves realigning and reactivating communication between the Yin and Yang organs, which are considered to be complementary forces in Traditional Chinese Medicine. The Yin organs are associated with more passive functions, such as storage and nourishment, while the Yang organs are associated with more active functions, such as movement and transformation. The organs are believed to work in harmony with one another, and disruptions to this harmony can lead to health issues.

By removing blockages in the meridians and restoring communication between the Yin and Yang organs, the Lymph-Chi Treatment can bring optimal balance, stability, and harmony throughout the body. This can improve overall health and wellbeing, as well as prevent or alleviate specific health issues.

In addition to addressing physical blockages, the Lymph-Chi Treatment also works to remove blockages in the metaphysical body, such as emotional and spiritual blockages. By addressing both physical and metaphysical blockages, the treatment takes a holistic approach to health and wellness, recognizing the interconnectivity of the body, mind, and spirit.

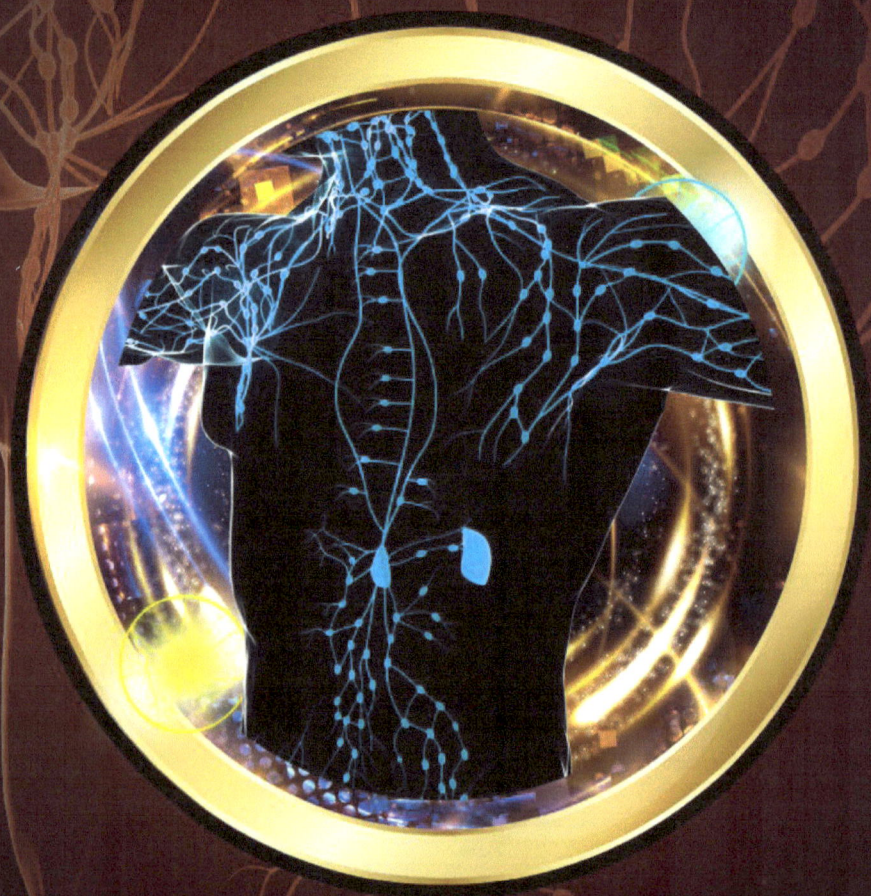

04

CONNECTION BETWEEN CHI AND THE LYMPHATIC SYSTEM

The life force energy flows through the body's organs, tissues, and cells and is responsible for maintaining health and vitality. According to TCM, blockages in the flow of Chi can cause physical and mental health problems, such as pain, fatigue, and emotional imbalances.

The lymphatic system, on the other hand, is responsible for filtering toxins and waste products from the body, as well as transporting white blood cells and other immune cells to fight infections and diseases. While the lymphatic system is a separate system from the meridians and the flow of Chi, some TCM practitioners believe that the lymphatic system and Chi are interconnected.

Blockages in the lymphatic system can cause a clutter of waste products in the body, which can then create blockages in the flow of Chi. In this way, lymphatic treatments, such as lighter touch or Lymph-Chi practices, may be used to help clear blockages in the flow of Chi and promote overall health and wellbeing.

Additionally, the blood and lymphatic systems work together to maintain overall health. The blood delivers oxygen and nutrients to the cells, while the lymphatic system removes waste and toxins. The two systems are interconnected, and imbalances in one system can affect the other. For example, a buildup of toxins in the lymphatic system can cause the blood to become thick and sluggish, leading to poor circulation and a variety of health problems.

By understanding the connection between Chi and the lymphatic system, as well as the relationship between the blood and lymphatic system, we can better appreciate the importance of maintaining a healthy flow of energy and waste removal in the body. Balancing and activating Chi, along with any other lymphatic treatment, can help promote optimal health and harmony in the mind, brain, body, and soul.

So, this section will explore the connection between Chi and the lymphatic system, understanding how balancing and activating Chi can bring harmony to the mind, body, and soul. We will also discuss the relationship between the blood and lymphatic system and how these two systems work together to maintain overall health and wellbeing.

Effects of Blockages in Chi on the Physical Body

In Traditional Chinese Medicine, the concept of Chi or life force energy is considered to be a vital force that flows throughout the body. This energy is believed to be responsible for the physical, mental, and emotional health of an individual. It is believed that when the flow of Chi is blocked, various physical and mental health problems can occur.

When there are blockages in the flow of Chi, it can lead to stagnation or a lack of circulation in certain areas of the body. This can cause a variety of physical symptoms, such as pain, stiffness, and tension. In some cases, it may also lead to the development of chronic conditions.

One of the primary ways in which blockages in Chi affect the physical body is by disrupting the balance and flow of vital energy through the meridians. Additionally, blockages in Chi can also affect the functioning of the internal organs. For example, if there is a blockage in Chi flow to the liver, it can lead to poor digestion, headaches, and fatigue. Similarly, blockages in Chi flow to the heart can cause chest pain, shortness of breath, and palpitations.

Over time, blockages in Chi can also lead to the development of chronic conditions, such as arthritis, hypertension, and diabetes. This is because when the flow of Chi is disrupted, it can lead to chronic inflammation and other changes in the body that can contribute to the development of these conditions.

In summary, the effects of blockages in Chi on the physical body can be significant and wide-ranging. By disrupting the flow of vital energy through the meridians and affecting the functioning of the internal organs, blockages in Chi can lead to a variety of physical and mental health problems, as well as the development of chronic conditions.

Balancing and Activating Chi Along with the Lymphatic System Brings Harmony to the Mind, Brain, Body, and Soul

Balancing and activating Chi, along with the lymphatic system, can bring harmony to the mind, brain, body, and soul. The lymphatic system is responsible for filtering toxins and waste from the body, while Chi is the vital energy that flows throughout the body. In Traditional Chinese Medicine, the lymphatic system is believed to play a role in the flow of Chi.

When the flow of Chi is disrupted, it can lead to physical and mental health problems. For example, blockages in Chi can cause stagnation, which can slow blood flow and manifest as various health issues. By restoring the free flow of Chi, the lymphatic system can work more effectively to filter out toxins and waste from the body, which can help prevent health problems.

When Chi and the lymphatic system are balanced and activated, the body can experience greater levels of harmony and wellbeing. This can lead to improved mental clarity, increased energy levels, and reduced stress and anxiety. The balanced flow of Chi can also help promote healthy sleep patterns, improve digestion, and enhance overall physical health.

In addition to improving physical health, balancing and activating Chi along with the lymphatic system can also have a positive impact on the mind and soul. Many people report feeling a greater sense of peace, calmness, and overall spiritual wellbeing after practicing techniques that promote the flow of Chi and lymph.

Some treatments that can be used to balance and activate Chi and the lymphatic system include acupuncture, acupressure, Qigong, Tai Chi, and herbal remedies. These practices work to stimulate the flow of Chi and encourage the lymphatic system to filter out toxins and waste from the body. By incorporating these practices into a daily routine, individuals can experience greater levels of harmony and wellbeing in their minds, body, and soul.

How to Protect the Body from Toxins

Although it's impossible to avoid all toxins, the human body is very resilient. This doesn't mean that you can engage in unhealthy behaviors, like chain-smoking or excessive drinking, without consequences. What it does mean is that our bodies have natural systems, like the lymphatic system, that help flush out toxins. As long as our exposure to toxins doesn't exceed our body's ability to eliminate them, our bodies can manage a certain amount of toxins. However, a higher toxic load can cause the body to work harder, which can take a toll in the long run. For example, although the liver is capable of metabolizing a lot of alcohol, years of excessive drinking can increase the risk of developing cirrhosis.

Since it's impossible to avoid all toxins, it's important to try to minimize your exposure to toxins as much as possible, both physically and mentally. To reduce toxic exposure, you can try eating organic foods whenever possible and avoiding artificial colors, flavors, and high fructose corn syrup. Everyone has at least one guilty pleasure that's not particularly healthy, but it's important to find a balance that works for you. For example, while some people might avoid gluten, wheat, salt, red meat, or caffeine, others might indulge in their favorite not-so-healthy snacks, like sour cream and onion potato chips.

You might not entirely exclude potato chips from your diet; however, eating them once a month isn't bad. That being said, be careful to choose a brand that is free of colors and artificial flavors.

However, it's important to note that not all toxins are eaten into the body. According to the Lymph-Chi practice, there are also energy toxins that can be felt in ways like bad emotions; hence, this should be eliminated at all costs.

Although our bodies can withstand a variety of emotions, it's crucial to let out unpleasant feelings as soon as they arise. Grief may become immobilized in the body and obstruct the Qi, or life force energy, from flowing freely when a person clutches onto it.

Moving physical substances through the body, such as blood through the circulatory system, food through the digestive system, and lymph via the lymphatic system, which aids in removing toxins, requires a smooth flow of Chi throughout the body.

Reducing Your Exposure to Toxins

The second guiding concept of decreasing your toxic load is customized to match your lifestyle and include your favorite activities. Here are three easy ways to lessen the total amount of toxins your body is exposed to:

Focus on reducing your overall toxin exposure

Living in a modern society means that it's impossible to avoid toxins entirely. However, instead of stressing out about trying to eliminate every single one, it's more productive to look at the overall amount of toxins you're exposed to throughout the week.

To get started, ask yourself these questions:

What am I drinking and eating?

How much pollution and chemicals am I being exposed to?

Am I experiencing high levels of stress?

What steps can I take to reduce overall exposure this week?

For example, if you're going through a particularly stressful week (which can result in emotional toxins), consider skipping alcoholic drinks when you're out with friends over the weekend. Alternatively, try to find a simple mocktail with no alcohol, or one that includes herbs, such as linden or even lavender mixed with alcohol-free sparkling wine.

Moreover, consider stress-reducing practices like yoga, guided imagery, meditation, deep breathing and body scanning. These practices will help reduce the body's production of cortisol as well as many other stress-production hormones, thus boosting the alignment of the physical with the metaphysical body.

Small changes first

One of the most significant obstacles to making changes is aiming for sudden and extreme change. Many diets are restrictive and leave you feeling deprived. For instance, if you want to stop eating pasta and bread, making this change overnight may be incredibly difficult to maintain, especially if these foods have been part of your diet for years. Instead, try starting small by reducing your intake and then gradually eliminating it over time. Continue to do this until it feels simple and effortless. Remember: Every small change tips the scale in your favor.

Locating The Chi Reflexology Points to Activate and Drain the Lymphatic System

The reflexology point is positioned on both feet in the webbing between the big toe and second toe, starting at the base of the toes and continuing to the point where the bones of these two toes meet, creating a V shape. Applying mild to medium pressure and pumping the area 15 times can help stimulate the lymphatic system; however, this approach should not be used as a substitute for physical movement and exercise. In conjunction with stimulating the primary reflexology points for the organs and meridians, regularly activating the lymphatic reflexology points can be an excellent starting point to improve lymphatic flow. It can also help clear energy blocks in the lymphatic system and increase the flow of Chi/Qi and lymph. Additionally, there are also reflexology points for the upper and lower lymph nodes.

Lymph-Chi Treatment for the Reflexology Point

Note: *If you are pregnant, please avoid massaging this point, as it overlaps with the acupressure point, liver 3, which is sometimes used in Eastern medicine to induce labor.*

Below are the instructions for lighter touch application on the reflexology point:

To apply light touch on the reflexology point, use the knuckle of your index finger to press and stroke the point. Place the knuckle at the base of the toes between the big toe and second toe, and then stroke down away from the toes and towards the point where the two bones meet in a *V*-shape.

When you reach the bottom of the *V*, lift your knuckle, reposition it at the base of the two toes, and repeat the downward stroke. It is essential to stroke only in one direction, away from the toes, as this correlates to the lymphatic flow throughout the body.

To apply the right amount of pressure, press down firmly enough to feel it but not so hard that it causes bruising or skin irritation. If the point is too sensitive, use lighter pressure. It is also recommended to use a lubricant, such as massage oil or moisturizer, to minimize friction and prevent skin irritation.

Calming the Reflexology Lymphatic System with Chi

- To apply light touch and acupressure therapy on the reflexology lymphatic point, start by doing 15 downward strokes on one foot and then repeat the same on the other foot. It is recommended to follow this routine twice a week.
- Avoid applying light touch on the reflexology point if you are pregnant, and do not exceed the recommended 15 strokes per foot twice a week.
- Over-massaging can irritate the skin or trigger detox symptoms if your body has a high level of toxins.

Apart from physical massages, it is equally important to let go of negative thoughts and behaviors that do not support your health and wellbeing. Chinese reflexology helps improve the flow of Qi through the area, but it is essential to keep the big picture in mind while detoxing. Remember not to overdo it, push yourself too hard, or want to fix yourself too quickly, as these can be counterproductive to your healing journey.

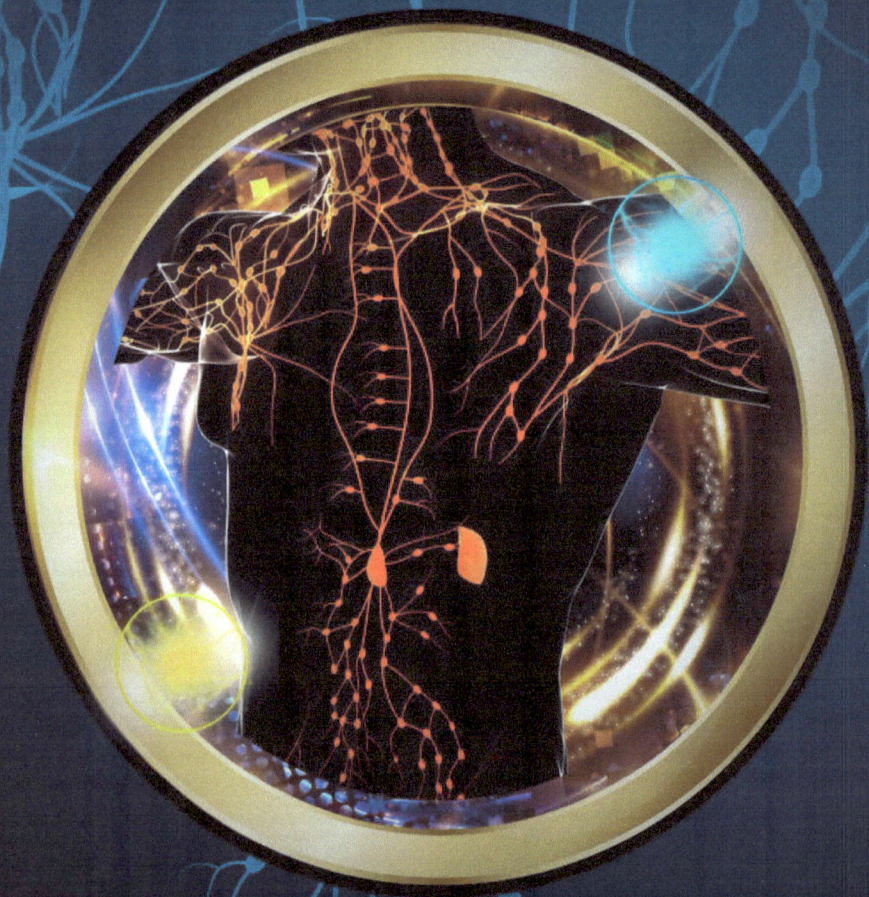

05

THE METAPHYSICAL BODY AND ITS EFFECT ON THE PHYSICAL BODY

The human body is a complex and intricate system that operates on multiple levels. While the physical body is what we can see and touch, there is also a deeper, metaphysical aspect that is often overlooked. The metaphysical body, also known as the energy body or aura, is composed of various energy centers or chakras and meridians or energy pathways. The health and wellbeing of the metaphysical body can have a profound effect on the physical body, influencing everything from disease and healing to mental and emotional states.

The concept of the metaphysical body has been an integral part of several ancient cultures and spiritual practices. It refers to the energy body that exists within and around the physical body and is responsible for maintaining the balance and flow of life force energy, also known as Qi, Prana, or Ki, depending on the tradition. This energy body is composed of several subtle energy channels, known as nadis, meridians, or chakras, depending on the culture.

In Traditional Chinese Medicine, the metaphysical body is known as the meridian system, which consists of a network of energy channels that run throughout the body and connect the organs and tissues. Similarly, in Ayurveda, the metaphysical body is composed of several chakras or energy centers that govern different aspects of physical, emotional, and spiritual health.

While the concept of the metaphysical body has been traditionally associated with spiritual and esoteric practices, modern research has begun to recognize the scientific basis of this concept. Studies have shown that the metaphysical body is closely connected with the nervous, endocrine, and immune systems of the body and plays a crucial role in maintaining overall health and wellbeing.

Therefore, exploring the connection between the metaphysical body and the lymphatic system is an important aspect of holistic health and wellness. In the following sections, we will explore the lymphatic system in detail and its relationship with the metaphysical body. We will also discuss the different ways in which we can optimize the health of both systems and promote overall vitality and longevity.

In this chapter, we will delve into the fascinating world of the metaphysical body and its relationship with the physical body. We will explore the intricate connection between these two aspects of the self and how understanding this connection can lead to greater health and wellness. We will discuss the connection between the metaphysical body and the lymphatic system, which plays a vital role in keeping our bodies healthy and functioning properly.

We will also examine how stress affects both Chi and the lymphatic system and the importance of balancing these systems for optimal health. Additionally, we will explore the role of the biomagnetic system, also known as the body's aura, in relation to the lymphatic system and overall health.

Moreover, we will delve into the effect of thought and emotions on the physical body and how they can manifest into physical symptoms. Finally, we will explore different metaphysical techniques and practices for balancing and strengthening the metaphysical body to promote optimal health and healing from specific illnesses. With a deeper understanding of the metaphysical body and its effects on the physical body, we can tap into our body's natural healing abilities and achieve a greater sense of wellbeing.

Chakras and Their Functions

Chakras are energy centers within the body that are believed to correspond to different physical, emotional, and spiritual aspects of the human experience. There are seven main chakras that are located along the central axis of the body, from the base of the spine to the crown of the head.

Each chakra is associated with a specific color, element, and sound, as well as specific physical and emotional functions. The seven chakras are as follows:

Root Chakra (Muladhara)

This is the first chakra in the body and is located at the base of the spine. It is associated with the color red, the element of earth, and the sound of "Lam." The root chakra governs our sense of safety, security, and stability.

When the root chakra is balanced and functioning properly, we feel grounded, secure, and stable in our lives. We are able to handle challenges and changes with a sense of ease and confidence. Physically, the root chakra is linked to the adrenal glands, which produce hormones that regulate our response to stress.

Imbalances in the root chakra can manifest as feelings of insecurity, fear, or anxiety, as well as physical symptoms, such as lower back pain, constipation, and issues with the legs, feet, or hips. A blocked root chakra can also lead to a lack of motivation or difficulty in making decisions.

There are several practices that can help balance the root chakra and promote a sense of grounding and stability. These practices include grounding exercises, such as walking barefoot on the earth or practicing yoga poses that focus on the lower body, such as the warrior series or tree pose. Meditation and visualization exercises that focus on the color red or the element of earth can also be helpful in balancing the root chakra.

It is important to note that the root chakra is interconnected with the other chakras, and imbalances in one chakra can impact the others. Therefore, it is important to approach chakra balancing as a holistic practice, addressing imbalances in all the chakras for optimal overall health and wellbeing.

Sacral Chakra (Svadhisthana)

The sacral chakra is often referred to as the center of creativity and pleasure. It is responsible for governing the emotions, sexual energy, and creativity in a person's life. The sacral chakra is associated with the color orange, which represents warmth, creativity, and passion.

In the physical body, the sacral chakra is linked to the reproductive system, bladder, and kidneys. Imbalances in this chakra can manifest in physical symptoms, such as sexual dysfunction, menstrual problems, or lower back pain.

Emotionally, a balanced sacral chakra allows individuals to express themselves creatively, have healthy relationships, and experience pleasure. However, when this chakra is blocked or imbalanced, individuals may experience a lack of creativity, sexual dysfunction, or feel emotionally stagnant.

Healing practices for the sacral chakra include movement-based practices like yoga or dance, meditation, journaling, and energy healing modalities, such as Reiki or chakra balancing. It is important to also address any underlying emotional or psychological issues that may be contributing to the blockage or imbalance of the sacral chakra.

Solar Plexus Chakra (Manipura)

The solar plexus chakra is located in the upper abdomen, just below the rib cage. This chakra is associated with the color yellow, which is often associated with the sun and warmth. The element of fire is also associated with this chakra, which represents transformation and the ability to take action.

The solar plexus chakra is responsible for our sense of personal power and self-confidence. When this chakra is balanced and flowing, we feel a sense of inner strength and the ability to take action toward our goals. We are confident in our decisions and feel a sense of purpose and direction in life.

However, when the solar plexus chakra is blocked or imbalanced, we may feel a lack of self-confidence and a fear of taking risks or making decisions. We may struggle with feelings of anxiety or insecurity and may feel a sense of powerlessness in our lives.

To balance the solar plexus chakra, practices such as yoga, meditation, and energy healing can be helpful. Specific yoga poses, such as boat pose, or warrior III, can help stimulate this chakra, while meditation and energy healing techniques can help release any blockages and restore the flow of energy. Additionally, incorporating yellow foods, such as bananas or yellow bell peppers into the diet can also help support the solar plexus chakra.

Heart Chakra (Anahata)

The heart chakra is the fourth chakra, located at the center of the chest. It is associated with the color green, the element of air, and the sound of "Yam." The heart chakra is the center of emotional wellbeing and is closely associated with the heart and lungs.

The heart chakra governs our ability to give and receive love, compassion, and forgiveness. When this chakra is in balance, we are able to love ourselves and others unconditionally, and we are able to form healthy, meaningful relationships. We are also able to feel empathy and compassion for others, and we are able to forgive ourselves and others for past mistakes.

When the heart chakra is blocked or imbalanced, we may experience emotional issues, such as jealousy, anger, and bitterness. We may also struggle with trust issues and find it difficult to form healthy relationships. Physical symptoms of an imbalanced heart chakra may include chest pain, heart palpitations, and difficulty breathing.

There are various practices that can help balance the heart chakra, including meditation, yoga, and energy healing. Engaging in acts of love and kindness, both towards ourselves and others, can also help open and balance this chakra. By doing so, we can experience greater emotional wellbeing, stronger relationships, and a deeper sense of love and compassion toward ourselves and others.

Throat Chakra (Vishuddha)

Also known as the Vishuddha, the throat chakra is located in the throat area and is associated with the color blue. This chakra is associated with the element of ether, also known as space, which represents the openness and expansiveness needed for clear communication. The sound associated with the throat chakra is "Ham," which is said to resonate with the vibrational frequency of this energy center.

The throat chakra is responsible for our ability to communicate effectively and authentically, both verbally and non-verbally. It governs all aspects of communication, including speaking, listening, and expressing ourselves creatively. When the throat chakra is in balance, we are able to express ourselves clearly and confidently, and we are able to listen to others with empathy and understanding.

However, when the throat chakra is blocked or imbalanced, we may experience difficulty in communication. This can manifest as fear of speaking, stuttering, or difficulty expressing ourselves creatively. We may also struggle with listening to others and understanding their point of view.

There are several techniques that can help balance the throat chakra and promote clear communication. These include chanting, singing, speaking affirmations, and practicing mindful listening. Additionally, using gemstones, such as blue lace agate or aquamarine, can help activate and balance the throat chakra, as can practicing yoga poses, such as the fish pose or the plow pose. By promoting balance and openness in the throat chakra, we can enhance our ability to communicate effectively and authentically, both with ourselves and with others.

Third Eye Chakra (Ajna)

The third eye chakra is located in the center of the forehead, between the eyebrows. It is associated with the color indigo and is often depicted as a lotus flower with two petals.

The third eye chakra is associated with our intuition, inner wisdom, and spiritual insight. It is believed to be the center of our psychic abilities, including clairvoyance, clairaudience, and telepathy. When this chakra is open and balanced, we are able to trust our inner guidance and have a deeper understanding of ourselves and the world around us.

However, if the third eye chakra is blocked or imbalanced, we may experience difficulties in trusting our intuition or making decisions. This can lead to feelings of confusion, disconnection, and lack of purpose.

There are various practices that can help balance the third eye chakra, including meditation, visualization, and yoga. Additionally, incorporating foods and herbs that support the health of the brain and nervous system, such as blueberries, walnuts, and ginkgo biloba, may also be beneficial.

It is important to note that while the third eye chakra is associated with spiritual insight, it is not meant to be a substitute for critical thinking or rational decision-making. Rather, it is a tool to enhance our overall awareness and understanding of ourselves and the world.

Crown Chakra (Sahasrara)

This chakra is located at the top of the head and is associated with the color violet or white, the element of thought, and the sound of silence. It is the highest chakra in the body and represents our connection to the divine, spiritual enlightenment, and higher consciousness.

The crown chakra is often depicted as a thousand-petaled lotus, representing the infinite nature of consciousness. It is the center of spiritual awareness, unity, and transcendence. When the crown chakra is open and balanced, we experience a deep sense of connection to the universe and a heightened sense of awareness.

Imbalances in the crown chakra can manifest as feelings of disconnection, lack of purpose, and spiritual emptiness. Physical symptoms can include headaches, insomnia, and sensitivity to light and sound. To balance the crown chakra, one can engage in practices that promote spiritual connection and self-awareness, such as meditation, prayer, and spending time in nature.

Through these practices, we can awaken and balance the energy of the crown chakra, allowing us to access our highest potential and connect with the divine. A balanced crown chakra can lead to a sense of purpose and meaning in life, spiritual fulfillment, and a deep understanding of the interconnectedness of all things.

In conclusion, according to the concept of the metaphysical body, each chakra is associated with specific physical organs, glandular systems, and emotional states. A balanced and unobstructed flow of energy through the chakras promotes optimal physical health, emotional wellbeing, and spiritual connection. Conversely, if the chakras are blocked or imbalanced, we may experience a range of physical, emotional, or spiritual symptoms.

Energy Flow and Blockages in the Metaphysical Body

Energy flow and blockages in the metaphysical body are central to the concept of chakras and the overall health of the body, mind, and spirit. The idea behind the metaphysical body is that there is an interconnectedness between the physical body, emotional state, and spiritual energy. This interconnectedness is believed to be regulated by energy centers called chakras, which are located along the spine.

Energy blockages in the chakras can disrupt the flow of energy throughout the body, leading to physical and emotional symptoms. As highlighted earlier, each chakra is linked to specific organs, glands, and body systems; this implies that an imbalance in one chakra can have a ripple effect throughout the body. For example, an imbalance in the root chakra, which is located at the base of the spine and is associated with feelings of safety and security, can lead to physical symptoms such as lower back pain or digestive issues.

Energy blockages can be caused by a variety of factors, including stress, trauma, negative thoughts, and beliefs. For instance, a traumatic experience can cause an energy blockage in the heart chakra, which is associated with love and compassion, leading to emotional symptoms like grief or heartache. Negative thoughts and beliefs can also contribute to energy blockages, as they can create energetic patterns that disrupt the flow of energy.

There are various practices that can help clear energy blockages and restore the flow of energy in the chakras. Meditation and yoga can help quiet the mind and bring awareness to the body, allowing for the release of blockages. Acupuncture can help stimulate the flow of energy through the body, while energy healing modalities, such as Reiki, can help remove blockages and restore balance to the chakras. By releasing these blockages, the energy flow can be restored, allowing the body, mind, and spirit to return to a state of balance and harmony.

Meditative State and How It Affects the Body

The meditative state can have a profound impact on the flow of Chi in the body. Meditation can help individuals achieve a more relaxed and focused state of mind, allowing for the free flow of Chi throughout the body.

During meditation, individuals often focus on their breath and become more aware of their body's sensations. This awareness can help them identify areas of tension or blockages in their energy pathways, allowing them to release those blockages and allow for the free flow of Chi.

In addition, meditation can help reduce stress and anxiety, which are known to impede the flow of Chi in the body. When the body is under stress, the muscles tense up, and the energy pathways can become blocked, resulting in a decreased flow of Chi. By reducing stress through meditation, the body can relax, and the energy pathways can open, allowing for the free flow of Chi.

Moreover, meditation can also improve one's mental state and emotional balance, which can positively impact the flow of Chi in the body. Negative emotions, such as anger, fear, and sadness, can cause blockages in the energy pathways, while positive emotions like joy and gratitude can enhance the flow of Chi.

Overall, the meditative state is an effective way to enhance the flow of Chi in the body. By reducing stress, improving emotional balance, and increasing awareness of the body's sensations, meditation can help individuals achieve a state of harmony and balance, allowing for the free flow of Chi throughout the body.

Connection Between the Metaphysical Body and the Lymphatic System

The metaphysical body and the lymphatic system may seem like two unrelated concepts, but in reality, they are closely connected. The metaphysical body is the non-physical aspect of our being that encompasses our emotions, thoughts, and spiritual nature. The lymphatic system, on the other hand, is responsible for the body's immune function, waste removal, and fluid balance.

In Eastern medical practice, the lymphatic system is believed to be connected to chakras in the body. Each chakra is associated with a specific area of the body and a specific set of emotions and thoughts. When the energy in a particular chakra is blocked or stagnant, it can affect the corresponding organ system and cause physical symptoms.

For example, the root chakra, located at the base of the spine, is associated with the lymphatic system and the immune system. When this chakra is out of balance or blocked, it can lead to immune dysfunction and an increased risk of infections. The sacral chakra, located just below the navel, is associated with the reproductive system and the lymphatic system. When this chakra is out of balance, it can lead to issues with the lymphatic system, including lymphedema.

The lymphatic system is also connected to the emotional body through its role in waste removal. The lymphatic system helps remove toxins and waste products from the body, including metabolic waste from cellular processes and environmental toxins. When the lymphatic system is not functioning properly, these waste products can build up and cause inflammation and other health issues. In the same way, when we hold onto negative emotions and thoughts, it can create an energetic blockage that can manifest as physical symptoms.

To maintain optimal health and balance in both the lymphatic system and the metaphysical body, it is important to take a holistic approach. Practices such as meditation, yoga, energy healing, light message massage, hydrotherapy, energy healing, and acupuncture can help clear blockages and promote the free flow of energy in the body. Additionally, maintaining a healthy lifestyle with a balanced diet, regular exercise, and adequate rest can help support the lymphatic system and the body as a whole.

Importance of Maintaining a Healthy Lymphatic System for Overall Metaphysical Health

From a metaphysical perspective, the lymphatic system is closely connected to the flow of energy throughout the body. Just as energy can become blocked or stagnant in the chakras, it can also become blocked or stagnant in the lymphatic system. When this happens, it can lead to a range of physical and emotional symptoms, including fatigue, pain, and a sense of being "stuck" or stagnant in life.

Maintaining a healthy lymphatic system is, therefore, essential for promoting overall metaphysical health. This can be achieved through a combination of lifestyle factors and holistic practices. Some key strategies for supporting lymphatic health include:

Exercise: Regular physical activity is essential for supporting lymphatic function. Exercise helps to stimulate the flow of lymphatic fluid through the body, which in turn helps to remove toxins and waste.

Hydration: Drinking plenty of water is essential for maintaining healthy lymphatic function. Water helps to flush toxins and waste out of the body, and it also helps to keep the lymphatic fluid flowing smoothly.

Nutrition: A healthy diet rich in fruits and vegetables can help to support lymphatic health by providing the body with essential nutrients and antioxidants. Foods that are high in fiber can also help to promote healthy bowel movements, which are important for lymphatic function.

Mind-body practices: Practices such as meditation, yoga, and deep breathing can help to support lymphatic health by reducing stress and promoting relaxation. When the body is in a state of relaxation, the lymphatic system can function more efficiently.

By taking care of our lymphatic system, we can support the flow of energy throughout the body and promote overall metaphysical health. By incorporating these strategies into our daily routine, we can help to keep our lymphatic system healthy and functioning optimally.

How Stress Affects Both Chi and the Lymphatic System

Stress can have a significant impact on both the flow of Chi in the metaphysical body and the functioning of the lymphatic system.

In terms of Chi, stress can cause blockages or disruptions in the flow of energy throughout the body. This can lead to physical and emotional symptoms, such as tension, pain, anxiety, and depression. When stress becomes chronic, it can also lead to more serious health problems, such as heart disease, high blood pressure, and autoimmune disorders. It is believed that stress affects the root chakra, which is associated with the lymphatic system and the immune system. When the root chakra is out of balance, it can lead to immune dysfunction and an increased risk of infections.

Stress can also have a direct impact on the lymphatic system, which, as previously discussed, is responsible for removing toxins, waste, and other unwanted substances from the body. When the body is under stress, the lymphatic system may not function as efficiently, leading to a buildup of toxins and waste in the body. This can lead to a variety of health problems, including inflammation, infections, and lymphedema.

Stress is a common experience in daily life, and it can have a significant impact on both the Chi and the lymphatic system. One of the ways stress affects the lymphatic system is by increasing the production of stress hormones, such as cortisol. These hormones can interfere with the normal functioning of the lymphatic system, reducing the flow of lymphatic fluid and impeding the removal of waste and toxins from the body. In turn, this can lead to a buildup of toxins and metabolic waste, which can impair the body's natural healing processes.

In addition, stress can also cause muscle tension, which can impede lymphatic flow and lead to lymphatic congestion. The lymphatic vessels rely on the contraction of smooth muscles to propel lymphatic fluid through the body, and tension in the muscles can interfere with this process. This can cause lymphatic fluid to accumulate in certain areas of the body, leading to swelling, discomfort, and an increased risk of infection.

To maintain healthy Chi and a healthy lymphatic system, it is important to manage stress levels through practices like meditation, yoga, deep breathing exercises, and regular exercise. These practices can help reduce stress, promote relaxation, and improve overall health and wellbeing. Additionally, maintaining a healthy diet, staying hydrated, and getting adequate sleep can also support the healthy functioning of both the metaphysical body and the lymphatic system.

In summary, stress can have a significant impact on both the Chi and the lymphatic system, and it is important to take steps to manage stress levels to support optimal health and wellbeing. By incorporating practices that promote relaxation, reduce muscle tension, and support lymphatic flow, individuals can maintain a healthy balance of energy and optimize their overall physical and metaphysical health.

Role of the Biomagnetic System (Body's Aura) In the Lymphatic System

The biomagnetic system, also known as the aura, is an electromagnetic field that surrounds the physical body. This field is made up of different layers, or subtle bodies, each of which corresponds to a different aspect of our being. These subtle bodies interact with the physical body, as well as with the environment around us.

The lymphatic system plays a crucial role in maintaining the health and wellbeing of the physical body. It is responsible for removing waste and toxins from the body, as well as supporting the immune system. The lymphatic system works in close connection with the circulatory system, which is responsible for circulating blood and nutrients throughout the body.

The biomagnetic field is believed to play a role in the functioning of the lymphatic system. The energy flowing through the biomagnetic field interacts with the lymphatic system, helping regulate lymphatic flow and supporting the removal of waste and toxins from the body.

When the biomagnetic field is healthy and balanced, it can support the functioning of the lymphatic system. However, when the biomagnetic field is disrupted or imbalanced, it can lead to lymphatic congestion and other issues.

There are many factors that can disrupt the biomagnetic field, including stress, illness, and environmental factors, such as electromagnetic radiation. When the biomagnetic field is disrupted, it can lead to a variety of physical, emotional, and spiritual symptoms.

The human body is surrounded by a biomagnetic field, also known as the aura, which is a complex energy field made up of electromagnetic energy. This field interacts with the environment and can be influenced by various internal and external factors, including emotional states, thought patterns, and environmental toxins. The health and balance of the biomagnetic field can play a significant role in the health and function of the lymphatic system.

The biomagnetic field is believed to contain seven layers, each corresponding to one of the chakras. These layers are thought to interpenetrate and influence one another, creating a dynamic energy field that surrounds and permeates the physical body. The health and balance of each layer of the biomagnetic field can impact the corresponding chakra and the organs, glands, and systems associated with it.

In addition to its relationship with the chakras, the biomagnetic field also interacts with the lymphatic system. The lymphatic system is responsible for removing waste and toxins from the body and plays a vital role in maintaining overall health and immunity. The flow of lymphatic fluid can be influenced by the health and balance of the biomagnetic field. When the biomagnetic field is disrupted, it can lead to blockages in the flow of lymphatic fluid, causing lymphatic congestion and increasing the risk of infections and other health issues.

To maintain a healthy biomagnetic field and support the healthy functioning of the lymphatic system, it is important to engage in practices that promote balance and wellbeing. Practices that promote relaxation and stress reduction, such as meditation, yoga, sound healing, going for a walk in nature, guided imagery, hypnotherapy or massage, can also support the health and balance of the biomagnetic field and promote healthy lymphatic flow.

It is also important to pay attention to environmental factors that can impact the biomagnetic field. Exposure to electromagnetic radiation from electronic devices or environmental toxins can disrupt the biomagnetic field and impede healthy lymphatic flow. By taking steps to reduce exposure to these factors and support the health and wellbeing of the biomagnetic field, we can support the healthy functioning of the lymphatic system and promote overall health and vitality.

The Effect of Thought and Emotions on the Physical Body

The mind-body connection is a well-established concept in many cultures and healing practices. It suggests that our thoughts and emotions can have a profound impact on our physical health and wellbeing. The concept of the mind-body connection suggests that our mental and emotional states can influence the functioning of our physical body and vice versa.

When we experience strong emotions or stressful situations, our body's stress response is triggered, which can lead to physiological changes, such as increased heart rate, shallow breathing, and muscle tension. Over time, these changes can lead to chronic health conditions, such as hypertension, cardiovascular disease, and chronic pain.

Negative emotions, such as anger, anxiety, and depression, have also been linked to an increased risk of developing chronic illnesses. For example, studies have shown that individuals with chronic pain who also have symptoms of depression or anxiety may experience more severe pain and a decreased response to pain medication.

On the other hand, positive emotions, such as happiness, gratitude, and love, have been shown to have numerous health benefits, including reducing stress levels, improving cardiovascular health, and boosting the immune system.

In addition to emotions, our thoughts and beliefs can also have an impact on our physical health. For example, individuals who hold negative beliefs about their health may be more likely to experience negative health outcomes than those who hold positive beliefs. This is because negative beliefs can lead to feelings of hopelessness and a lack of motivation to take care of one's health.

It is important to note that the mind-body connection is not a one-way street. Our physical health can also impact our mental and emotional wellbeing. Chronic pain or illness, for example, can lead to feelings of depression, anxiety, and stress.

In summary, our thoughts and emotions can have a powerful impact on our physical health and wellbeing. It is important to cultivate positive emotions and beliefs, manage stress, and take care of our physical health to promote overall health and vitality.

Realigning Your Chi

There are several techniques to control Chi, since it plays a part in every bodily function. If you have healthy breathing, eating, and sleeping habits, your prognosis for Chi will probably be favorable. Some claim that if you don't perform these three things, your Chi won't be able to flow properly, and you'll likely keep having trouble with whatever health issue you're experiencing.

To control your Chi, it is essential to stay away from harmful interactions. We all have those people in our lives who drain the Chi. After speaking with them, you feel physically drained and exhausted; that's because they have sapped your Chi. And then there are those who boost your confidence and energize you. That Chi exchange is positive and essentially needed.

However, your Chi is vital, not just for healing and staying fit but for overall daily activity, and that is why you need to guard it diligently. To ensure you keep your Chi in check, there are a few things you can do to help regulate your Chi and how you channel it over time. These include but are not limited to getting enough restful sleep, exercising often, especially breathing exercises like yoga, keeping good eating routines, and taking care of your emotional health.

Rest well

When it comes to balancing your Chi and preventing a Chi deficit, getting enough restful sleep and living at a slower pace are both essential. A chronic lack of restful sleep can lead to fatigue and a further imbalance of the body's energy. It is recommended that adults aim for seven to nine hours of sleep each night to promote restorative rest.

In addition to getting enough sleep, it is also important to live at a slower pace and avoid constantly being on the go. Multitasking should be minimized as much as possible, and breaks should be taken throughout the day to rest and recharge.

Practices such as meditation, deep breathing, and mindfulness can also be helpful in slowing down and finding inner peace. By taking the time to pause, reflect, and connect with the present moment, individuals can better align their Chi and promote overall balance and harmony in the body, mind, and spirit.

Practice breathing

Through deliberate breathing, a Chi deficiency can be remedied. If you find it difficult to breathe deeply, you may be anxious, which may result in a Chi shortage.

You may practice a variety of breathing techniques to balance your Chi. Diaphragmatic breathing, often known as belly breathing, is one technique. Either reclining or standing up is acceptable. This is how it goes:

- Inhale slowly and deeply via your nose.
- Visualize your stomach expanding as you take a breath in.
- Permit that breath to fill up your stomach. Your abs should be relaxed. (Place your palm on your stomach; at this point, you should feel your stomach swell slightly).
- Breathe out through your mouth.

Qigong or Tai Chi

Gentle exercises, such as Tai Chi and Qigong, can be an effective way to control and balance one's Chi. These two martial arts have been practiced for centuries and have been shown to have a range of benefits for both physical and mental health.

Individuals of all ages and fitness levels can perform Tai Chi, as it has been shown to improve balance, flexibility, and muscle strength. Tai Chi has also been linked to a reduction in stress and anxiety, as well as improvements in cognitive function and overall quality of life.

Qigong, on the other hand, has been shown to have a range of benefits, including improved cardiovascular health, reduced stress and anxiety, improved joint mobility, and relief of chronic pain.

Regular practice of these gentle exercises can help prevent sickness and maintain overall health and wellbeing. By balancing and regulating the flow of Chi in the body, individuals may experience improved immune function, reduced inflammation, and a lower risk of developing chronic illnesses. Additionally, the mental and emotional benefits of these exercises can help promote a sense of inner peace and harmony, leading to a greater sense of overall wellbeing.

Maintain a balanced diet

Having a balanced, nutrient-rich diet is an essential aspect of maintaining balanced Chi. The food we consume provides the majority of the body's Chi, making it vital to nourish our bodies with nutritious foods that support a healthy digestive system and promote healing. In Chinese medicine, food is viewed as medicine, and choosing the right types of food can help balance and regulate the flow of energy in the body.

One common nutritional therapy for balancing Chi is to avoid cold meals, raw foods, fried foods, dairy products, and junk food. Instead, it is recommended to steam, grill, or roast meals, as these therapeutic approaches help preserve the food's nutrients and energy. Warming foods, such as chicken, ginger, whole grains, bamboo, and mushrooms, are also beneficial for balancing Chi.

As you choose the right types of food, it is essential to eat mindfully and in moderation. Overeating can lead to imbalances in the digestive system and disrupt the flow of Chi in the body. It is recommended to eat slowly, chew food thoroughly, and stop eating when you feel full.

Overall, here are some foods that can enhance Lymph-Chi:

Leafy Greens: Dark, leafy greens like spinach, kale, and collard greens are rich in antioxidants and nutrients that can help support lymphatic function. In addition to their antioxidant and nutrient content, dark, leafy greens are also rich in chlorophyll, a powerful detoxifying agent that can help support the body's lymphatic system. The lymphatic system plays a critical role in removing toxins and waste from the body, and by eating foods like spinach, kale, and collard greens, you can help support the function of this important system.

Furthermore, leafy greens are particularly beneficial for healing and supporting the liver, which is a key organ in the body's detoxification process. The liver plays a critical role in filtering out toxins and waste products from the blood, and by consuming leafy greens regularly, you can help keep this vital organ functioning optimally.

Also, leafy greens are also beneficial for supporting the cardiovascular system. They contain compounds that can help improve blood flow and reduce inflammation in the arteries, which can help lower the risk of heart disease.

Finally, leafy greens are an excellent source of fiber, which is important for maintaining a healthy digestive system. By promoting regular bowel movements and supporting the growth of beneficial gut bacteria, fiber can help prevent a variety of digestive issues, including constipation and bloating.

Citrus Fruits: Citrus fruits like oranges, grapefruits, and lemons are high in vitamin C, which can help boost the immune system and support lymphatic health. Citrus fruits are rich in bioflavonoids, which help enhance the absorption of vitamin C and strengthen the immune system. Bioflavonoids also act as antioxidants and anti-inflammatory agents, protecting cells from damage caused by free radicals and reducing inflammation throughout the body.

In addition to boosting the immune system, vitamin C also plays a critical role in maintaining the health of the lymphatic system. The lymphatic system relies on vitamin C to produce lymphocytes, which are specialized white blood cells that help fight infections and diseases. Without sufficient levels of vitamin C, the lymphatic system may not be able to function properly, leading to a weakened immune system and a higher risk of illness.

Consuming citrus fruits regularly can also help promote healthy skin and reduce the risk of skin diseases. Vitamin C is a vital nutrient for collagen synthesis, which is essential for maintaining skin elasticity and preventing skin damage caused by free radicals. Citrus fruits also contain limonoids, which are compounds that have been shown to have anti-cancer properties and may help prevent the development of certain types of cancer, including skin cancer.

Garlic: Garlic has antibacterial and anti-inflammatory properties that can help boost the immune system and reduce inflammation in the body. It contains a compound called allicin, which gives it its characteristic pungent smell and has potent antimicrobial effects. Garlic has long been regarded as a potent natural remedy for various health conditions, including its ability to purify the Chi. Garlic contains potent antibacterial and anti-inflammatory properties that help boost the immune system and reduce inflammation in the body. By reducing inflammation, the body can better eliminate toxins and other harmful substances that can interfere with the flow of Chi.

Garlic is also known to contain sulfur compounds that help detoxify the body by supporting the liver's natural cleansing process. These compounds help break down harmful toxins in the liver and facilitate their removal from the body, resulting in a healthier flow of Chi.

Furthermore, garlic has a warming nature that helps increase circulation and promote the energy flow throughout the body. This helps restore balance to the body's energy systems, which can help reduce fatigue and improve overall wellbeing. By including garlic in your diet, you can purify your Chi and support your body's natural healing processes.

Ginger: Ginger has anti-inflammatory and antioxidant properties that can help support lymphatic function and reduce inflammation. Ginger has been shown to have a number of health benefits that can help enhance the body's Chi and promote healing, especially during post-operative recovery. Its anti-inflammatory properties can help reduce swelling and inflammation, which can be particularly beneficial for individuals recovering from surgery.

In addition, ginger's antioxidant properties can help protect the body against damage from free radicals, which are unstable molecules that can cause cellular damage and contribute to the development of chronic diseases. By reducing oxidative stress in the body, ginger can help promote overall health and wellbeing.

Furthermore, ginger has been found to have immune-boosting properties, which can be especially helpful during post-operative recovery when the body is more vulnerable to infections. By supporting the immune system, ginger can help the body fight off harmful pathogens and promote faster recovery.

Finally, ginger can help support lymphatic function by promoting circulation and reducing congestion in the lymphatic system. By improving lymphatic flow, ginger can help enhance the body's natural detoxification processes and support overall health and wellbeing.

Turmeric: Turmeric contains curcumin, which has anti-inflammatory and antioxidant properties that can help support lymphatic health. Turmeric is a spice commonly used in Indian and Middle Eastern cuisine. It contains curcumin, a powerful antioxidant that has anti-inflammatory properties and has been used for centuries in Ayurvedic and Chinese medicine to treat a variety of ailments.

Studies have shown that curcumin can help reduce inflammation in the body and may even have anti-cancer properties. It is also believed to help support lymphatic health by reducing swelling and improving circulation.

In terms of enhancing the body's Chi for healing and post-operative recovery, turmeric may help reduce pain and inflammation after surgery or injury, allowing the body to heal more efficiently. Additionally, its anti-inflammatory properties may help prevent scar tissue formation and improve overall recovery time.

Incorporating turmeric into your diet is easy; it can be used in a variety of dishes, from curries to soups to smoothies. You can also take turmeric supplements in capsule form, although it's always best to consult with a healthcare provider before starting any new supplement regimen.

Berries: Berries like blueberries, strawberries, and raspberries are high in antioxidants and can help support lymphatic function. Berries are not only delicious but also a great source of nutrients that can help promote lymphatic function and enhance the body's Chi for healing and post-operative recovery. These fruits are rich in antioxidants, particularly anthocyanins, which help protect the body from free radicals that can damage cells and lead to inflammation. Antioxidants also help boost the immune system, which is essential for overall health and wellness.

Berries are particularly beneficial for post-operative recovery because they contain anti-inflammatory properties that can help reduce swelling and promote healing. After surgery, the lymphatic system may be impaired, leading to a buildup of fluids in the body that can cause discomfort and slow down the healing process. Eating berries can help support lymphatic function, allowing the body to remove excess fluids and toxins from the body efficiently.

Additionally, berries are rich in fiber, which can help support digestive health and promote regular bowel movements. This is particularly important after surgery, as pain medication and anesthesia can slow down the digestive system and lead to constipation. Consuming berries can help keep the digestive system healthy and functioning properly, allowing the body to absorb nutrients more effectively.

Incorporating berries into your diet is easy and delicious. They can be eaten as a snack or added to smoothies, salads, or yogurt. By consuming a variety of berries regularly, you can help promote lymphatic function, reduce inflammation, and enhance the body's Chi for optimal healing.

Bone Broth: Bone broth is rich in collagen and amino acids that can help support lymphatic health and boost the immune system. Bone broth has gained popularity as a health-boosting beverage in recent years, and it is a great source of essential nutrients for the lymphatic system. Collagen and amino acids present in bone broth help promote healthy connective tissue throughout the body. This connective tissue is crucial for lymphatic function since it provides a structure that allows the lymphatic fluid to flow through the body.

Bone broth is also high in minerals like calcium, magnesium, and phosphorus, which help support overall bone health. Additionally, the nutrients in bone broth have been shown to have anti-inflammatory properties, making it an excellent option for those recovering from surgeries or injuries.

The amino acid glycine found in bone broth can help support liver function, which is critical for maintaining a healthy lymphatic system. The liver plays a vital role in filtering toxins from the body, and a healthy liver is essential for optimal lymphatic function.

Nuts and Seeds: Nuts and seeds like almonds, walnuts, and chia seeds are high in healthy fats and nutrients that can help support lymphatic function. Nuts and seeds are great sources of healthy fats and nutrients that can help support lymphatic function, which is crucial for the proper functioning of the immune system. Almonds, for instance, are rich in vitamin E, which is a powerful antioxidant that helps protect the body against cellular damage and inflammation. Walnuts are a good source of omega-3 fatty acids, which are anti-inflammatory and may help reduce the risk of chronic diseases, such as heart disease and cancer.

Chia seeds are another great addition to a healthy diet to support lymphatic function. They are a good source of fiber, protein, and omega-3 fatty acids. The fiber in chia seeds helps promote healthy digestion and elimination, which is important for removing waste products and toxins from the body. Additionally, chia seeds are rich in antioxidants, which can help protect the body against cellular damage and inflammation.

Adding nuts and seeds to your diet can help improve post-operative recovery, as they provide the body with important nutrients that help support the immune system and reduce inflammation. Additionally, the healthy fats in nuts and seeds can help the body absorb fat-soluble vitamins such as vitamins A, D, E, and K, which are crucial for overall health and wellbeing.

Maintaining Mental Wellness

The mind-body connection plays a significant role in the balance of one's Chi. If your mental health isn't in check, it can lead to an imbalance in your body's energy levels. Therefore, it is essential to maintain good mental health as well as physical health. If you experience anxiety or depression, seeking therapy from a mental health expert can be helpful. They can provide you with the necessary support and tools to manage your mental health effectively.

Other things you can do to boost your lymphatic system and Chi include various practices, such as massage, body scrubs, colonics, chiropractic, and acupressure, all of which have been proven to promote relaxation, overall calmness, reduce stress, and improve mood. Exercises, such as yoga, Tai Chi, or Qigong, can also be helpful in managing mental health. These practices not only help in calming the mind but also promote the circulation of energy throughout the body, resulting in a sense of balance and harmony.

Maintaining strong and positive social connections is also crucial for good mental health. Loneliness can result in harmful physical symptoms, such as increased inflammation and higher levels of stress hormones. Therefore, it is essential to maintain good relationships with family, friends, and loved ones. Participating in group activities or volunteering can also help in maintaining social connections and promoting a sense of belonging.

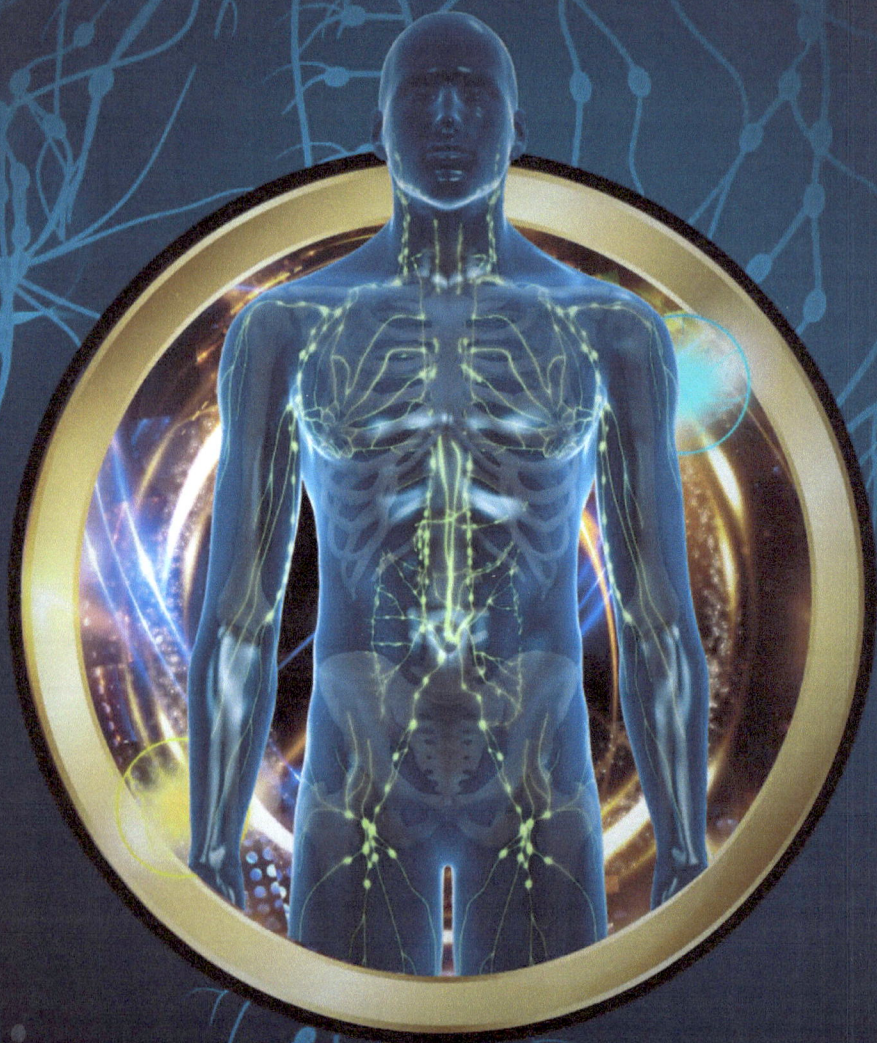

06

HOW THE LYMPH-CHI TREATMENT WORKS

The lymphatic system and the concept of Chi, or life force energy, have been foundational components of traditional healing practices for centuries. Both systems are recognized for their critical role in promoting optimal health, supporting the immune system, and removing waste and toxins from the body. The Lymph-Chi Treatment is a holistic approach that combines the principles of these two systems to promote balance, harmony, and healing in the body. By integrating techniques from both systems, the Lymph-Chi Treatment offers a unique and powerful healing modality that can support overall health and wellbeing. In this chapter, we will explore the principles behind the Lymph-Chi Treatment, the techniques used, and the benefits that can be achieved through this transformative approach to healing.

Understanding the Physiology of Lymph-Chi

By combining these two approaches (Western and Eastern medicine), the Lymph-Chi Treatment offers a comprehensive and effective way to support the body's natural healing processes. By following the lymphatic system through the body and draining the built-up fluids and toxins out of the body, this treatment promotes optimal healthy functioning of the lymphatic system, which is essential for overall wellness.

In addition to the physical benefits, the Lymph-Chi Treatment can also have a positive impact on mental and emotional wellbeing. By reducing stress and anxiety, this treatment can help individuals feel more grounded, centered, and at ease. Improved sleep and breathing patterns can lead to greater relaxation and a sense of calm, which can also support mental and emotional wellness.

Furthermore, rebalancing the mind-brain-body-spirit-soul connection is a key aspect of the Lymph-Chi Treatment. This holistic approach recognizes the interconnectedness of all aspects of the self and works to bring balance and harmony to the entire being. By promoting this balance, individuals may experience a greater sense of clarity, purpose, and overall wellbeing.

This treatment offers a comprehensive approach to health and healing that can support individuals in achieving optimal physical, mental, emotional, and spiritual wellbeing. Its combination of Eastern and Western healing practices, along with its focus on the lymphatic system and life force energy, makes it a unique and powerful approach to holistic health.

The Lymph-Chi Treatment is a powerful tool for promoting overall health and wellness. By understanding the physiology behind this treatment and how it works, individuals can harness its full potential for healing and rejuvenation.

Ideally, it focuses on following the lymphatic system through the body and using specific techniques to drain built-up fluids and toxins out of the body. By doing so, it promotes the healthy functioning of the lymphatic system, which can lead to overall wellness and vitality.

This treatment can be particularly effective in post-operative recovery, as it promotes the body's natural healing processes and can help reduce swelling and inflammation. It can also be used to reduce stress and anxiety, improve sleep, and promote healthy breathing patterns.

Some Medical Conditions Lymph-Chi Helps Treat

The combination of Lymph-Chi and the principles of Chi can be a powerful tool in the treatment of various medical conditions. Here are some examples:

Chronic Fatigue Syndrome

Chronic Fatigue Syndrome (CFS) is a condition that can be debilitating for those who suffer from it. It is a complex condition characterized by persistent fatigue that is not relieved by rest. CFS can also cause symptoms such as headaches, joint pain, and difficulty concentrating. While the exact cause of CFS is not known, there are many theories that suggest it may be linked to immune system dysfunction or viral infections.

Lymph-Chi Treatment can be a useful therapy option for those with CFS. This therapy can help boost the immune system and reduce inflammation in the body. Light touches can help stimulate the lymphatic system, which is responsible for removing toxins and waste from the body.

In addition to Lymph-Chi, the principles of Chi can also be helpful in treating CFS. The Chinese belief is that CFS can be a result of a blockage of Chi energy in the body. By using techniques such as acupuncture, acupressure, or Qigong, the flow of energy can be restored to the body. This can help increase energy levels and reduce fatigue.

Furthermore, mindfulness techniques, such as meditation, can also be helpful in managing the symptoms of CFS. By practicing mindfulness, individuals can learn to be more present, reduce stress and anxiety, and improve their overall wellbeing.

Ultimately, a combination of Lymph-Chi Treatment, mindfulness, and other complementary therapies can be an effective treatment option for those with chronic fatigue syndrome. It can help to reduce inflammation, boost the immune system, restore balance and energy flow in the body, and improve overall wellbeing.

Fibromyalgia

Fibromyalgia is characterized by chronic pain, stiffness, and tenderness in the muscles and soft tissues of the body, often accompanied by fatigue, headaches, and sleep disturbances. While the exact cause of fibromyalgia is unknown, it is believed to be related to abnormal pain processing in the central nervous system, which amplifies painful sensations throughout the body.

Lymph-Chi Treatment can be a valuable tool for managing fibromyalgia symptoms. Lymph-Chi can help reduce pain and inflammation by promoting the drainage of excess fluids and toxins from the affected tissues. By reducing inflammation, the therapy can also help improve mobility and range of motion in affected joints.

Moreover, the principles of Chi can help restore balance and energy flow to the body, which is crucial in managing fibromyalgia symptoms. The therapy can improve circulation and oxygenation of the affected tissues, which can alleviate pain and stiffness. The deep breathing exercises and meditative practices associated with the therapy can also help reduce stress and improve mental clarity, which is important in managing the emotional and cognitive aspects of fibromyalgia.

Furthermore, Lymph-Chi Treatment can be used in conjunction with other treatments for fibromyalgia, such as medication and physical therapy. By integrating different approaches, clients can achieve a holistic and comprehensive treatment plan that addresses their specific needs and goals. Ultimately, Lymph-Chi Treatment can improve the quality of life for people with fibromyalgia by reducing pain and improving physical and emotional wellbeing.

Lymphedema

Lymphedema is characterized by the accumulation of lymphatic fluid in the tissues, which can cause swelling, discomfort, and reduced mobility. Lymph-Chi Treatment can be an effective treatment for lymphedema, as it can improve lymphatic flow and reduce inflammation in the affected area.

Lymph-Chi can help manually stimulate the lymphatic system and encourage the flow of lymphatic fluid, which can help reduce swelling and promote healing. This therapy can include compression bandaging and exercise therapy to encourage movement of the affected limb.

The principles of Chi can also be beneficial in treating lymphedema, as they can help improve circulation and promote the flow of energy through the affected area. This can be achieved through techniques such as acupressure, Qigong, and meditation.

In addition to manual therapy and energy-based techniques, lifestyle changes can also play an important role in managing lymphedema. This can include maintaining a healthy weight, exercising regularly, and avoiding activities that may exacerbate swelling.

Ultimately, by promoting lymphatic flow and improving energy circulation, Lymph-Chi Treatment can reduce swelling, alleviate discomfort, and improve the overall quality of life for those with lymphedema.

Arthritis

Arthritis is a prevalent condition that affects millions of people worldwide, and it can significantly impact the quality of life of those who suffer from it. Arthritis causes pain, stiffness, and inflammation in the joints, making it challenging to carry out daily activities, such as walking, lifting objects, or even holding a pen.

Lymph-Chi Treatment is a non-invasive and natural approach that can help alleviate the symptoms of arthritis. By combining light touches and the principles of Chi, it is possible to promote healing and improve the overall health of the joints.

The principles of Chi can also play a vital role in the treatment of arthritis. By promoting the flow of energy in the body, Chi can improve circulation and promote healing. When the energy is blocked, it can cause pain and stiffness in the joints, exacerbating the symptoms of arthritis. By using Chi-based techniques, such as acupuncture or acupressure, it is possible to release these blockages and improve the flow of energy to the affected areas.

Furthermore, Lymph-Chi Treatment can also help improve overall physical and mental wellbeing. By reducing pain and inflammation in the joints, it is possible to improve mobility and reduce the risk of falls, which can lead to fractures and other injuries. Additionally, by promoting relaxation and reducing stress, Lymph-Chi Treatment can improve sleep, mood, and overall quality of life.

Depression and Anxiety

Depression and anxiety are two of the most common mental health conditions that can affect a person's quality of life. These conditions can manifest in different ways, such as persistent sadness, loss of interest, nervousness, or restlessness. In severe cases, depression and anxiety can interfere with a person's ability to carry out their daily activities, affecting their personal and professional relationships.

Lymph-Chi can be helpful in treating depression and anxiety by promoting relaxation and reducing stress. By stimulating the lymphatic system, lymphatic gentle touch therapy helps release toxins from the body and reduce inflammation, which can contribute to feelings of stress and anxiety. The gentle and rhythmic massage strokes used in Lymph-Chi can also help calm the nervous system, promote relaxation, and improve sleep quality.

In addition to Lymph-Chi, the principles of Chi can also be beneficial in treating depression and anxiety. According to Traditional Chinese Medicine, imbalances in the flow of Chi can contribute to emotional and mental disturbances. By balancing the flow of energy in the body, the principles of Chi can help restore a sense of emotional and mental equilibrium, promoting a sense of wellbeing and reducing symptoms of depression and anxiety.

To integrate the principles of Chi into the treatment of depression and anxiety, various techniques can be used, including acupuncture, acupressure, and herbal remedies. Acupuncture involves the insertion of fine needles into specific points on the body to balance the flow of Chi. Acupressure, on the other hand, involves applying pressure to specific points on the body using the fingers or other instruments. Both techniques can help reduce stress and promote relaxation.

Herbal remedies can also be used to support the treatment of depression and anxiety. Certain herbs have been traditionally used in Chinese medicine to help balance emotions and promote a sense of calm, such as St. John's Wort and valerian root. It is important to consult a trained practitioner to determine the most appropriate herbal remedies for each individual's needs and health history.

Insomnia

Insomnia is a common sleep disorder that affects people of all ages, genders, and backgrounds. It can be caused by various factors, such as stress, anxiety, physical discomfort, or even certain medications. Insomnia can have a negative impact on one's overall health and wellbeing, affecting their ability to function during the day, leading to mood swings, lack of focus, and even physical fatigue.

Lymph-Chi can be an effective treatment option for insomnia, as it can help reduce stress and promote relaxation. This therapy involves the use of gentle touch therapy to stimulate the lymphatic system and promote the flow of lymph fluid throughout the body. By doing so, Lymph-Chi can help flush out toxins and waste products from the body, reducing inflammation and promoting a sense of calmness.

In addition to Lymph-Chi, the principles of Chi can also be helpful in treating insomnia. In Chinese medicine, it is believed that an imbalance in Chi can cause disruptions in sleep patterns. By restoring balance to the body's energy flow, Chi can promote restful sleep and improve overall sleep quality.

Practices such as acupuncture, Qigong, and meditation can all be helpful in promoting healthy Chi flow and improving sleep patterns. Meditation can also be effective in promoting relaxation and reducing stress levels, which can, in turn, improve sleep patterns. If you are struggling with insomnia, consider exploring these treatment options with a qualified practitioner to find relief and improve your quality of life.

Digestive issues

From bloating to constipation and even more serious conditions like Irritable Bowel Syndrome (IBS) and acid reflux, these issues can be a source of discomfort and pain. Fortunately, Lymph-Chi Treatment can offer relief and support for individuals suffering from digestive issues.

Lymph-Chi can help reduce inflammation in the gut, which can be a major contributor to digestive issues. By improving lymphatic flow, Lymph-Chi can support the body's natural detoxification processes, helping eliminate toxins that may be causing inflammation. In addition, Lymph-Chi can improve circulation in the gut, which can promote healing and reduce discomfort.

The principles of Chi can also play a significant role in improving digestion and promoting a healthy gut microbiome. Chi energy can be used to stimulate specific acupressure points in the body that are connected to the digestive system. By activating these points, Chi energy can improve digestion and promote the movement of food through the digestive tract. In addition, Chi energy can be used to promote the growth of healthy gut bacteria, which can further support digestive health.

It is also worth noting that Lymph-Chi Treatment can be effective in addressing the root causes of digestive issues, including stress and anxiety. By reducing stress and promoting relaxation, Lymph-Chi and Chi energy can alleviate tension in the gut, leading to improved digestion and a reduction in symptoms.

Migraines

Migraines can be triggered by a variety of factors, including stress, changes in sleep patterns, hormonal changes, and certain foods. The pain of a migraine can be intense and may be accompanied by other symptoms, such as sensitivity to light and sound, nausea, and vomiting.

Lymph-Chi can be beneficial in the treatment of migraines by reducing inflammation in the body. When inflammation is present in the body, it can trigger a cascade of events that lead to migraines. By reducing inflammation, Lymph-Chi can help prevent migraines from occurring.

In addition to reducing inflammation, the principles of Chi can also be helpful in the treatment of migraines. By improving circulation and reducing stress, the body is better able to regulate its systems, which can help to prevent migraines. One study found that acupuncture, which is based on the principles of Chi, was effective in reducing the frequency and severity of migraines in participants.

It's important to note that migraines can have many underlying causes, and a combination of therapies may be needed for effective treatment. However, Lymph-Chi and the principles of Chi can be a valuable part of a comprehensive treatment plan for migraines. By reducing inflammation, improving circulation, and reducing stress, these therapies can both prevent and manage the symptoms of migraines, leading to a better quality of life for those who suffer from this condition.

Post-operative recovery

Lymph-Chi treatment can also be beneficial in post-operative recovery. After surgery, the body's natural healing process can be slow and painful. Swelling and inflammation are common, and it can take weeks or even months to recover fully. Lymph-Chi Treatment can help speed up the recovery process by increasing blood and lymphatic circulation, which can reduce inflammation and promote tissue regeneration.

The gentle movements and breathing techniques used in Lymph-Chi Treatment can also help alleviate stress and anxiety, which are common emotions experienced after surgery. Additionally, Lymph-Chi Treatment can improve the body's immune system function, which is crucial for post-operative recovery. By boosting the immune system, the body can fight off infections and heal faster.

It is important to note that Lymph-Chi Treatment should not be used as a substitute for medical treatment after surgery. However, when used in combination with medical treatment, it can help enhance the healing process and improve overall wellness. Consult your healthcare provider to determine whether Lymph-Chi Treatment is a safe and effective option for your post-operative recovery.

Lymph-Chi and enhancement of digestive health post-surgery

Undergoing surgery can take a toll on the body, and the recovery process involves not only healing the surgical site but also restoring the body's overall balance and function. One aspect of post-surgical recovery that is often overlooked is digestive health. The lymphatic system plays a crucial role in maintaining a healthy digestive system by removing waste, toxins, and excess fluid. However, below are some of the ways Lymph-Chi Treatment can help improve the digestive health during post-operative recovery:

Enhancing nutrient absorption

After surgery, the body may struggle to absorb nutrients efficiently, leading to malnutrition and weakened overall health. The lymphatic system plays a crucial role in transporting nutrients from the digestive system to the bloodstream. Lymph-Chi Treatment can enhance lymphatic circulation, thereby improving nutrient absorption in the small intestine. By optimizing nutrient uptake, Lymph-Chi Treatment supports the body in obtaining the necessary building blocks for healing and recovery.

Reduces tendencies of constipation

Constipation is a common issue following surgery, often due to medications, changes in mobility, and dietary alterations. Lymph-Chi Treatment can help alleviate constipation by stimulating peristalsis, the wave-like muscle contractions that move food through the digestive tract. Additionally, Lymph-Chi Treatment supports the elimination of waste products by improving lymphatic flow, thereby promoting regular bowel movements and relieving constipation.

Generally, the idea of Lymph-Chi is to enhance your wellbeing and improve your recovery speed from both simple and complex medical conditions by improving circulation, reducing inflammation, and restoring balance to the body's energy systems. Lymph-Chi and Chi principles can help promote healing and improve overall wellness.

How the Lymph-Chi Treatment Unblocks Channels and Lymphatic Flow Through the Body

One of the key components of the Lymph-Chi Treatment is its ability to unblock channels and restore the flow of lymphatic fluids through the body. In this section, we will explore how the treatment accomplishes this important goal.

The lymphatic system is a network of vessels, nodes, and organs that work together to remove waste and toxins from the body and support the immune system. When this system becomes blocked or compromised, it can result in a variety of health issues, including inflammation, infection, and chronic disease. The Lymph-Chi Treatment focuses on unblocking these channels and restoring the flow of lymphatic fluids to promote optimal health.

One of the key techniques used in the Lymph-Chi Treatment is light touch movement. This technique involves applying gentle pressure and rhythmic movements to specific areas of the body to stimulate the lymphatic system and encourage the flow of lymphatic fluids, therefore removing waste and toxins from the body and reducing inflammation and swelling.

In addition to light touches, the Lymph-Chi Treatment also incorporates acupressure techniques. These techniques involve applying pressure to specific points along the body's meridian lines to promote the flow of energy and unblock any areas of stagnation. This can help improve the flow of lymphatic fluids and support the body's natural healing processes.

Another key component of the Lymph-Chi Treatment is the use of herbal remedies and supplements. These natural remedies can help support the body's lymphatic system and promote optimal health. For example, herbs such as red clover and cleavers have been traditionally used to improve lymphatic function.

Overall, the Lymph-Chi Treatment offers a holistic approach to unblocking channels and restoring the flow of lymphatic fluids through the body. By incorporating techniques such as light touch, acupressure, and herbal remedies, this treatment can help promote optimal health and wellbeing by supporting the body's natural healing processes.

How Chi Flows into the Internal Organs

Ideally, with respect to the Lymph-Chi Treatment, we see the organs as not just anatomical structures but also as energetic systems that are closely related to our emotions, mental states, and overall health. This understanding is based on the concept of Chi, which flows throughout the body and is responsible for maintaining health and vitality.

When Chi is flowing smoothly, it can reach every part of the body, including the internal organs. Each organ is associated with a specific type of Chi, and an imbalance or blockage in this Chi can lead to health problems.

The liver, for example, is associated with the energy of anger and the emotion of frustration. When the liver Chi is blocked or imbalanced, it can manifest as symptoms such as headaches, mood swings, and digestive issues. The heart is associated with joy and happiness, and an imbalance in the heart Chi can lead to symptoms like palpitations and anxiety.

The lungs are associated with grief, and an imbalance in the lung Chi can manifest as shortness of breath and sadness. The kidneys are associated with fear, and an imbalance in the kidney Chi can lead to low back pain and urinary issues.

Understanding how Chi flows into the internal organs is crucial for maintaining good health and preventing illness. That being said, there are several ways to ensure that Chi is flowing smoothly into the internal organs. One of the most effective is through practices such as Tai Chi and Qigong, both of which can help balance and regulate the flow of Chi throughout the body.

In addition, acupuncture and other forms of Traditional Chinese Medicine can be used to help address imbalances in the organ systems and restore the flow of Chi. A healthy diet, regular exercise, and stress reduction techniques, such as meditation and yoga, can also be helpful in maintaining the free flow of Chi throughout the body.

The Science Behind the Treatment

The Lymph-Chi Treatment is a holistic approach that integrates both Eastern and Western schools of thought to promote balance, harmony, and healing in the body. The treatment is based on the principles of Traditional Chinese Medicine and the Western understanding of the lymphatic system. The lymphatic system is a complex network of vessels, nodes, and organs that work together to remove waste and toxins from the body, support the immune system, and promote optimal health.

In TCM, the concept of Chi or life force energy is central to understanding health and wellbeing. According to TCM, Chi flows through the body through channels known as meridians. When the flow of Chi is disrupted or blocked, it can lead to physical and emotional imbalances and illnesses.

The Lymph-Chi Treatment works to unblock channels and promote the free flow of lymphatic fluid and Chi through the body. This is achieved through various techniques, such as acupressure and deep breathing exercises. These techniques help stimulate the lymphatic system, improve circulation, and promote the flow of Chi through the body's meridians.

There is evidence to support the effectiveness of the Lymph-Chi Treatment. Light touches can reduce swelling in clients with lymphedema. Acupressure has also been shown to have therapeutic effects on various health conditions, including chronic pain, anxiety, and depression. Deep breathing exercises have been shown to promote relaxation and reduce stress.

Techniques and Practices for Balancing and Strengthening the Metaphysical Body to Promote Optimal Health and Healing

The metaphysical body, which includes the chakras, aura, and other energetic systems, plays a crucial role in our overall health and wellbeing. When these systems are out of balance or weakened, it can lead to physical, emotional, and spiritual imbalances. Fortunately, there are a variety of techniques and practices that can be used to balance and strengthen the metaphysical body and promote optimal health and healing.

Energy healing practices

Energy healing practices are based on the principle that the human body has an energy system responsible for maintaining physical, emotional, and mental health. When the energy flow is disrupted, it can lead to physical, emotional, and mental imbalances. Energy healing practices use various techniques to restore the balance of energy in the body and promote overall health and wellbeing.

Reiki is a popular energy healing practice that involves the use of hands-on or distant healing to balance the energy in the body. The practitioner channels universal energy through their hands to the client, promoting relaxation, reducing stress, and restoring balance to the energy system. Reiki has been found to be effective in reducing pain, anxiety, and depression, therefore improving overall wellbeing.

Crystal healing is a practice that involves the use of crystals and gemstones to restore balance to the body's energy system. Crystals and gemstones are believed to have unique properties that can help absorb negative energy, promote positive energy flow, and restore balance to the body's energy system. They can be used in various ways, such as wearing them as jewelry, placing them on specific points on the body, or carrying them in a pocket.

In addition to these energy healing practices, there are other techniques that can be used to balance and strengthen the metaphysical body. These may include practices such as yoga, Tai Chi, Qigong, and meditation. These practices work by promoting relaxation, reducing stress, and restoring balance to the energy system. It is important to work with a qualified practitioner when using energy healing practices to ensure safe and effective treatment.

Chakra balancing

Chakra balancing is a technique that has been used for centuries to promote balance and harmony in the body's energy systems. It involves working with the seven main chakras, which are located along the spine, to balance and align them. When the chakras are in balance, energy can flow freely through the body, supporting overall health and wellbeing.

There are many different ways to balance the chakras, and each individual may find certain treatments to be more effective than others. Some common techniques include visualization exercises, meditation, and energy healing practices, such as Reiki.

Visualization exercises involve using mental imagery to focus on each chakra, imagining it as a spinning wheel of energy. By visualizing the chakra spinning smoothly and evenly, we can help balance and align it. This technique can be done on its own or as part of a guided meditation.

Meditation is another powerful technique for chakra balancing. By focusing on the breath and bringing awareness to each chakra, we can release blockages and promote the free flow of energy through the body. There are many guided meditations available online that are specifically designed for chakra balancing.

Energy healing practices, such as Reiki, acupressure or acupuncture, can also be effective for chakra balancing. These techniques involve working with the body's energy systems to clear blockages and promote the free flow of energy. During a Reiki or acupuncture session, the practitioner will focus on specific points in the body, corresponding to the chakras, to promote balance and harmony.

In addition to these techniques, there are also many other practices that can support the healthy functioning of the chakras. These may include yoga, aromatherapy, and sound healing, among others. By incorporating these practices into our daily routine, we can promote balance and harmony in the body's energy systems, supporting overall health and wellbeing.

Meditation and mindfulness

Meditation and mindfulness practices have been used for centuries to promote inner peace, reduce stress, and improve overall wellbeing. These practices involve training the mind to focus on the present, which can reduce anxiety and increase feelings of calmness and relaxation.

There are many different types of meditation and mindfulness practices, each with their own unique techniques and approaches. Some common types of meditation include:

- **Mindfulness meditation:** This type of meditation involves paying attention to the present moment without judgment or distraction. It can be practiced in a seated position, while walking, or during daily activities.

- **Transcendental meditation:** This type of meditation involves repeating a mantra or sound to help quiet the mind and promote relaxation.
- **Loving-kindness meditation:** This type of meditation involves cultivating feelings of love, kindness, and compassion towards oneself and others.
- **Body scan meditation:** This type of meditation involves scanning the body from head to toe, noticing any sensations or areas of tension.

By practicing meditation and mindfulness regularly, we can train our minds to be more present, calm, and focused. This can help reduce stress and anxiety, improve sleep quality, and promote overall physical and emotional wellbeing.

In addition to formal meditation practices, there are also many mindfulness techniques that can be incorporated into daily life. These may include:

- **Deep breathing exercises:** Taking deep, slow breaths can reduce stress and promote relaxation.
- **Mindful eating:** Paying attention to the tastes, smells, and textures of food can promote mindful eating and reduce overeating.
- **Body awareness:** Paying attention to physical sensations and movements throughout the day can promote mindfulness and reduce stress.

Overall, incorporating meditation and mindfulness practices into daily life can be a powerful tool for supporting the health and wellbeing of the metaphysical body. By training the mind to be more present and focused, we can reduce stress and promote overall physical, emotional, and spiritual health.

Yoga

Yoga is an ancient practice that has been used for thousands of years to promote physical, mental, and spiritual health. It is a comprehensive system that combines physical postures, breathing exercises, and meditation to help balance and strengthen the body, mind, and spirit.

The physical postures, known as asanas, are designed to promote flexibility, strength, and balance in the body. Each posture targets different areas of the body, and many are specifically designed to stimulate and balance the chakras. For example, poses such as the tree pose (Vrikshasana) and warrior II pose (Virabhadrasana II) are believed to stimulate and balance the root chakra, while poses like the cobra pose (Bhujangasana) and bow pose (Dhanurasana) are believed to stimulate and balance the heart chakra.

Breathing exercises, known as pranayama, are also an important part of yoga practice. They help regulate the breath and calm the mind, which can reduce stress and promote relaxation. Some pranayama techniques are also believed to stimulate and balance the chakras. For example, alternate nostril breathing (Nadi Shodhana) is believed to stimulate and balance the third eye and crown chakras, while Kapalabhati breathing is believed to stimulate and balance the solar plexus chakra.

Sound healing

Sound healing is a holistic practice that has been used for thousands of years to promote physical, emotional, and spiritual healing. It involves the use of sound frequencies to create a state of deep relaxation and promote a sense of wellbeing. The sound frequencies used in sound healing are believed to correspond to specific chakras, and by working with these frequencies, we can balance and strengthen the metaphysical body.

One popular sound healing practice is listening to music or chants that are specifically designed to promote relaxation and healing. These sounds are often created using specific frequencies that are believed to have a beneficial effect on the body and mind. For example, the 528Hz frequency is known as the "love frequency" and is believed to promote feelings of love and wellbeing.

Another popular sound healing practice is the use of sound bowls. These bowls are made of various materials, such as crystal or metal, and produce a deep, resonant sound when struck or played. Each bowl is believed to correspond to a specific chakra, and by working with these bowls, we can help balance and strengthen the corresponding chakra.

Sound healing can also be used in conjunction with other practices, such as meditation or yoga. By incorporating sound into these practices, we can deepen our state of relaxation and promote a sense of inner peace and wellbeing. Sound healing can also be used as a stand-alone practice to promote relaxation and reduce stress.

Overall, sound healing is a powerful tool for balancing and strengthening the metaphysical body. By working with sound frequencies and vibrations, we can promote relaxation, reduce stress, and promote a sense of wellbeing and balance in our lives.

Mind-body techniques

Mind-body techniques are powerful tools that can promote balance and wellbeing in the metaphysical body. These practices involve harnessing the power of the mind to positively influence the body's physical and emotional responses.

Biofeedback is a technique that involves using sensors to monitor the body's physiological responses, such as heart rate and muscle tension. The feedback provided by the sensors can help individuals learn how to control these responses, promoting relaxation and stress reduction consciously. Biofeedback has been shown to be effective in treating a variety of physical and mental health conditions, including chronic pain, anxiety, and high blood pressure.

Hypnotherapy is a technique that involves inducing a state of deep relaxation and focused concentration to access the subconscious mind. This state of deep relaxation can be used to help individuals release emotional and physical tension, promote healing, and reduce stress. Hypnotherapy has been shown to be effective in treating a variety of conditions, including anxiety, phobias, and chronic pain.

Other mind-body techniques that can be used to support the healthy functioning of the metaphysical body include guided imagery, progressive muscle relaxation, and cognitive-behavioral therapy. These techniques can help individuals learn how to consciously influence their thoughts, emotions, and physical responses, promoting relaxation, stress reduction, and overall wellbeing.

Aromatherapy and essential oils

Aromatherapy is a holistic healing practice that involves the use of essential oils to promote physical, emotional, and spiritual wellbeing. Essential oils are highly concentrated plant extracts that contain the natural aroma and therapeutic properties of the plant. These oils can be used in a variety of ways, including diffusing them into the air, adding them to bathwater, or applying them topically to the skin.

For example, lavender essential oil is believed to promote relaxation and reduce stress, while frankincense essential oil is believed to promote spiritual wellbeing.

When it comes to balancing and strengthening the metaphysical body, aromatherapy can be a powerful tool. Different essential oils have different properties and can be used to support specific chakras or areas of the body. For example, lavender essential oil is known for its calming properties and can be used to balance the third eye chakra and promote spiritual insight. Peppermint essential oil is invigorating and can be used to stimulate the root chakra and promote physical energy and vitality.

To use essential oils for balancing and strengthening the metaphysical body, it is important to choose high-quality oils and use them safely. Essential oils are potent and can be harmful if not used properly. It is important to dilute essential oils in a carrier oil, such as coconut oil, before applying them to the skin and to avoid ingesting essential oils unless under the guidance of a trained professional.

One popular way to use essential oils for balancing the metaphysical body is through diffusing. By diffusing essential oils into the air, they can be inhaled and absorbed through the respiratory system, providing benefits to the entire body. For example, diffusing frankincense essential oil can promote spiritual awareness and balance the crown chakra while diffusing lemon essential oil can promote mental clarity and balance the solar plexus chakra.

Another way to use essential oils for balancing the metaphysical body is through massage. By adding essential oils to a carrier oil and massaging them into the skin, they can be absorbed through the skin and provide localized benefits. For example, massaging ginger essential oil into the lower abdomen can stimulate the sacral chakra and promote healthy sexual function, while massaging eucalyptus essential oil into the chest can promote respiratory health and balance the heart chakra.

Overall, aromatherapy and essential oils can be a powerful tool for balancing and strengthening the metaphysical body. By choosing high-quality oils, using them safely, and incorporating them into a holistic healing practice, we can support the health and wellbeing of the entire body, mind, and spirit.

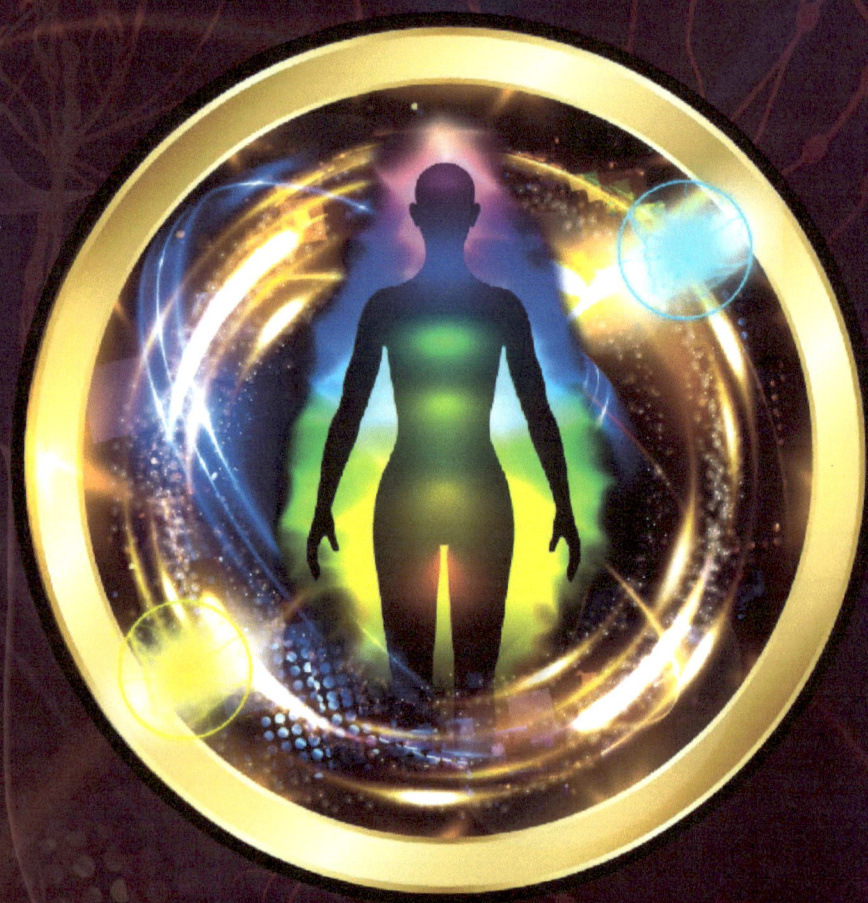

07

THYMUS GLAND AND THE DIRECT IMPACT OF LYMPH-CHI TREATMENT

Quite obviously, the dysfunctionality of one part of the body affects the proper operation of the other. However, the lymphatic system, a complex network of veins, organs, and tissues, maintains our body's general health and wellbeing. It oversees fluid homeostasis, immune system performance, and the body's elimination of waste and pollutants. The thymus gland, which plays a vital role in the lymphatic system's operation, is one of its often-disregarded parts.

In this chapter, we explore the lymphatic system's vast effects and how the thymus gland and other direct lymphatic organs affect the proper functionality of the body. We will analyze the complex interaction between the thymus gland and Chi, and how Lymph-Chi can help in maintaining balance in your system. We'll also learn how interference with the Chi flow and lymphatic system can prevent organs from communicating with one another, resulting in fatigue, weight problems, hormone imbalances, and more.

We will also learn the huge consequences that the thymus gland may have on our physical, emotional, and mental health. Generally, we will begin to understand the relevance of these elements when they are functioning effectively by looking at the activities of the thymus gland and other organs directly connected to the lymphatic system.

We'll also look into the interesting field of Lymph-Chi treatment in restoring normal organ function, encouraging weight control, hormone balance, and general wellbeing by treating dysfunctions and harmonizing the thymus gland.

This chapter will not only explain how the lymphatic system and the thymus gland are related, but will also outline useful methods for everyday thymus gland stimulation. Along with Lymph-Chi Treatment, these methods, such as tapping, stroking in a clockwise direction, and applying pressure, are simple to include in our regular activities. Let's get started,

Direct Organs of the Lymphatic System

The lymphatic system consists of several organs that work together to maintain fluid balance, support the immune system, and facilitate the removal of waste and toxins from the body.

Moreover, the lymphatic system is interconnected with various organs and tissues in the body, allowing for communication and coordination. It interacts with the circulatory system, as lymphatic vessels transport lymph and eventually return it to the bloodstream. The immune system relies on the lymphatic system for the transportation of immune cells, facilitating their surveillance and response to infections and diseases. Additionally, the lymphatic system communicates with other organ systems, such as the respiratory system (tonsils and adenoids) and the digestive system (Peyer's patches), to protect against pathogens entering through these routes.

Understanding the functions of these organs provides insight into the importance of a healthy lymphatic system. Here are the key organs of the lymph system:

- Lymph node
- Thymus

- Lymphatic vessel
- Spleen
- Right lymphatic duct
- Tonsil
- Adenoid
- Peyer's Patches
- Thoracic duct

Lymph nodes: These are small, bean-shaped structures scattered throughout the body and connected by lymphatic vessels. They act as filters, trapping harmful substances like bacteria, viruses, and abnormal cells. Lymph nodes contain immune cells that help fight infections and play a crucial role in the immune response.

Emotional and mental stress, negative thoughts, and physical factors, such as toxins and poor lifestyle habits, can adversely affect the function of the lymph nodes, which could lead to a reduced immune response and increased susceptibility to infections.

However, the Lymph-Chi Treatment helps address blockages within lymph nodes, restoring their optimal filtration capacity and enhancing immune system function.

Thymus: The thymus gland is a primary lymphatic organ located in the upper chest behind the sternum. It plays a vital role in the development and maturation of T lymphocytes, a type of white blood cell involved in immune system defense. The thymus gland is particularly active during childhood and gradually decreases in size with age.

Balanced Chi flow positively influences the thymus gland's ability to produce and mature T cells, promoting a robust immune response. However, toxins and hormonal imbalances can negatively affect the proper function of this gland function, leading to increased vulnerability to infections.

Lymphatic vessels: Lymphatic vessels form an extensive network throughout the body, similar to blood vessels. They carry lymph, a clear fluid containing waste products, excess fluid, and immune cells, from the tissues back to the bloodstream. Lymphatic vessels transport lymph to the lymph nodes, where it is filtered and purified before returning to the circulatory system.

Factors like poor circulation or inflammation can impede lymphatic flow, leading to fluid retention, toxin buildup, and compromised immune responses. However, Lymph-Chi treatment enhances the opening and clearing of lymphatic vessels, facilitating the smooth flow of lymph fluid, enhancing detoxification, and supporting immune system health.

Spleen: This is the largest lymphatic organ and is located in the upper left abdomen. It acts as a filter for the blood, removing old or damaged red blood cells, bacteria, and other foreign substances. The spleen also plays a role in immune responses by producing antibodies and storing immune cells.

When the Chi is balanced, it helps ensure the spleen works optimally for blood purification and immune responses.

Chronic inflammation or compromised circulation can impact spleen function, leading to reduced blood filtration and weakened immune defenses.

However, Lymph-Chi Treatment helps fix blockages within the spleen, restoring its optimal filtering capacity, enhancing immune system function, and promoting overall vitality.

Right lymphatic duct: This is a small duct that collects lymph from the right side of the head, neck, and upper limb, as well as the right side of the thorax. It drains into the right subclavian vein, returning lymph to the bloodstream.

A balance in Chi guarantees an efficient drainage of lymphatic fluid through the right lymphatic duct, aiding in fluid balance and immune responses.

Emotional stress, physical trauma or injury, and postural imbalances can impact the flow of lymphatic fluid through the right lymphatic duct, leading to fluid retention and compromised immune functions. However, Lymph-Chi Treatment helps in ensuring the smooth drainage of lymphatic fluid and supporting immune system health.

Tonsils: There are small masses of lymphatic tissue located at the back of the throat. They help trap and eliminate pathogens that enter the body through the mouth and nose, acting as a defense mechanism against infections.

Adenoid: Also known as the pharyngeal tonsil, this is a mass of lymphatic tissue located at the back of the nasal cavity. Similar to the tonsils, it helps protect against infections by trapping and eliminating pathogens.

Peyer's patches: There are clusters of lymphatic tissue found in the small intestine, primarily in the ileum. They play a crucial role in monitoring and responding to intestinal pathogens, contributing to the immune defense in the digestive system.

When the Chi functions optimally with no blockages, it enhances the ability of the tonsils, adenoids, and Peyer's patches to trap and eliminate pathogens.

Factors like chronic respiratory infections and poor digestive health can affect the performance of tonsils, adenoids, and Peyer's patches, compromising their ability to defend against pathogens.

However, the Lymph-Chi Treatment helps with removing blockages within these lymphatic tissues, revitalizing their function and enhancing effective immune responses.

Thoracic duct: This is the largest lymphatic vessel in the body. It collects lymph from the lower body, the left side of the head and neck, and the left upper limb. The thoracic duct then drains into the left subclavian vein, returning lymph to the bloodstream.

A balanced Chi will help in maintaining fluid balance and supporting immune responses. Emotional stress, physical trauma or injury, and postural imbalances can impact the flow of lymphatic fluid through the thoracic duct, leading to fluid retention and further collapse of the immune system. Lymph-Chi Treatment will help in ensuring the smooth drainage of lymphatic fluid and supporting immune system health.

Evidently, each of these organs has a unique role in the lymphatic system's overall function. Blockages within the lymphatic system or disruptions in Chi flow can hinder the communication and optimal performance of these organs, leading to various health issues. Lymph-Chi Treatment addresses these dysfunctions, allowing for rebalancing and revitalizing the organs of the lymphatic system.

Impact of Blockages on the Interaction of the Organs

Blockages in the lymphatic system and disrupted Chi flow can have a significant impact on the communication between the organs of the lymphatic system and the rest of the body. When blockages occur within this system or when Chi flow is disrupted, several consequences can arise, hindering effective communication and coordination between these organs and the rest of the body.

Impaired fluid balance

The lymphatic system plays a crucial role in maintaining fluid balance within the body. It helps remove excess fluid, waste products, and toxins from the tissues. Blockages in the lymphatic vessels can lead to fluid retention, swelling (edema), and impaired fluid circulation. This can disrupt the exchange of nutrients, oxygen, and waste products between organs, impeding their normal functioning.

Low immune response

The lymphatic system is intricately linked to the immune system. Lymph nodes, thymus, spleen, and other lymphatic organs are essential for immune cell production, activation, and immune response coordination. When blockages occur in the lymphatic vessels or when Chi flow is disrupted, the transportation of immune cells and communication between lymphatic organs and the immune system may be hindered. This can lead to a weakened immune response, making the body more susceptible to infections and diseases.

Inhibited detoxification

Blockages in the lymphatic vessels can impede the efficient drainage of waste products, resulting in toxin buildup and impaired detoxification processes. This can impact the overall health and functioning of organs and systems, leading to various health issues.

Cloaked communication and signaling

The organs of the lymphatic system, such as lymph nodes, spleen, and thymus, communicate with other organs and tissues in the body through the release of chemical messengers, immune cells, and lymphatic fluid. When blockages or disrupted

Chi flow occurs, the communication pathways may be compromised, hindering the exchange of signals, nutrients, and information between these organs and other body systems. This can disrupt the coordination of physiological processes and compromise overall health.

In this light, the aim of the Lymph-Chi Treatment is to remove obstacles to communication within the lymphatic system and between the lymphatic system and other organs. By promoting efficient fluid circulation, immune response, detoxification, and inter-organ communication, Lymph-Chi Treatment helps promote the optimal functioning of the lymphatic system and its coordination with the rest of the body for overall vitality.

The Thymus Gland and the Immune System Development

The wellbeing and maintenance of the immune system depend on a number of organs that make up the lymphatic system. The thymus gland, which is the main lymphatic organ, plays an integral part among these organs. The red bone marrow and the thymus gland are the two main lymphatic organs, which should be noted before going into more detail about the thymus.

The production of different blood cells, including immune cells like lymphocytes, is carried out by the red bone marrow, which is largely present in the long bones and flat bones of the body. It is the location where they mature and differentiate, and it is very important for the early phases of immune cell formation.

The red bone marrow's activities are supplemented by the thymus gland, which is situated in the chest above the heart. It is very important throughout childhood and adolescence, gradually becoming smaller and less active as you become older. T lymphocytes, sometimes referred to as T cells, are a particular kind of lymphocyte that form and mature in the thymus gland.

T cells are important immune system actors because they can identify and attack certain infections and aberrant cells. They coordinate and control a number of immune system functions, including other immune cells' activation and operation. T cells may develop in the thymus gland, where they can also go through a process of instruction and selection. It guarantees that T cells acquire the capacity to differentiate between self and non-self, limiting autoimmune responses and fostering a powerful immune response against invading foreign invaders.

T cells in the thymus interact with specialized cells known as thymic epithelial cells throughout the maturation process and receive signals that mold their functional features. This complex process is supported by the distinct milieu that the thymus offers, enabling T cells to develop the broad repertoire required to identify a variety of infections and abnormalities.

The thymus is essential for the growth of the immune system, but as we become older, it becomes less active. T cell maturation and production therefore decline, which influences immune system performance. This loss is thought to be a factor in elderly people's greater vulnerability to infections and diminished immune surveillance.

The necessity of preserving the thymus gland's optimum function is highlighted by knowledge of the gland's role in immune system growth and maintenance. Lymph-Chi Treatment may assist in the rejuvenation of the thymus gland, boosting T cell maturation and the general effectiveness of the immune system by eliminating obstructions and fostering balanced Chi flow.

Importance of the Thymus Gland for the Overall Function of the Lymphatic System

The thymus gland is essential to how the lymphatic system functions as a whole. While the lymphatic system is in charge of the growth and development of T cells, other organs within the system also play significant roles in maintaining a strong immune response. One such organ is the liver, which is responsible for several metabolic activities and is also the body's main producer of lymph.

The lymphatic system plays a crucial role in the formation and operation of the liver. Lymph, a fluid produced from interstitial fluid, is discharged from the liver tissue through a network of lymphatic veins. Numerous items, including immune cells, proteins, waste materials, and other things, are present in this lymph. To keep the liver healthy and the immune system functioning properly, the lymphatic veins of the liver are essential.

It's interesting to note that a process known as lymph angiogenesis has been associated with an increase in the number of hepatic lymphatic vessels in a variety of liver illnesses, including cirrhosis, viral hepatitis, and hepatocellular carcinoma. It is believed that this angiogenesis, or the growth of new lymphatic vessels, is a reaction to the underlying disease alterations taking place in the liver. It is thought to help remove toxins, cellular debris, and inflammatory mediators from the liver tissue as part of the body's effort to manage the illness.

The importance of lymph angiogenesis in liver disorders emphasizes how closely the lymphatic system and the liver are connected. The lymphatic veins in the liver support immunological response and surveillance in addition to helping with waste product removal. They aid in the movement of immune cells to and from the liver tissue, including lymphocytes, dendritic cells, and macrophages, aiding immune defense and controlling inflammation.

The intricate relationship between lymphatic function and organ health is highlighted by an understanding of how the liver's lymphatic system is involved in different liver disorders. Immune performance, waste clearance, and general liver health may all be impacted by any disturbances or abnormalities in the lymphatic system of the liver. Therefore, keeping a healthy lymphatic system is crucial for promoting immunological responses, detoxification procedures, and general wellbeing. This includes the lymphatic veins of the liver operating properly.

By resolving obstructions and fostering balanced Chi flow within the liver's lymphatic system, Lymph-Chi Treatment may promote the organ's healthy operation. Lymph-Chi Treatment may help improve immune responses and promote the removal of waste products and toxins, helping the liver as well as the whole body by improving lymphatic circulation and the general health of the lymphatic system.

Chi and Its Association with the Thymus Gland

Chi has a substantial impact on the harmony and vitality of the lymphatic system within the context of the thymus gland. The thymus gland and the heart meridian, which are both regarded to be the main channels through which Chi flows, according to Eastern medicine, are closely related. The heart meridian is in charge of transporting Chi throughout the body and promoting maximum performance. The thymus gland's vitality and general health are directly impacted by the flow of Chi since it is connected to the heart meridian.

The thymus gland performs better when Chi is flowing easily and harmoniously. Consequently, the immune system's reaction to infections and abnormalities is strengthened as a result of the maturation and growth of T cells. To preserve the health of the immune system and improve the body's capacity to fight off illnesses, the thymus gland's ability to channel Chi in a balanced manner is essential.

The thymus gland and the whole lymphatic system, on the other hand, may be impacted by Chi blockages or disturbances. The thymus gland's capacity to operate at its peak might be hampered when Chi becomes sluggish or insufficient. Immunological system function may be disrupted, mature T cell generation may be reduced, and immunological response abnormalities may result.

The movement of Chi inside the thymus gland and the lymphatic system may also be influenced by emotions, ideas, and physical conditions. The thymus gland's vitality and its function in the control of the immune system may be impacted by emotional stress, unfavorable ideas, and bad lifestyle choices. This can disturb the harmonious flow of Chi. The proper operation of the thymus gland and the general health of the lymphatic system, on the other hand, may be supported by happy emotions, a tranquil mind, and healthy lifestyle choices.

These obstructions and imbalances in the lymphatic system and thymus gland's Chi flow are treated by Lymph-Chi Treatment. Lymph-Chi Treatment works to revitalize the thymus gland and promote the balance and vitality of the lymphatic system by using methods like tapping, rubbing, and applying pressure to certain locations.

The body's self-healing processes may be triggered by Lymph-Chi Treatment, assisting in clearing obstructions, reestablishing energy balance, and supporting the thymus gland's healthy operation. This improves the lymphatic system's general effectiveness, enhancing immunological responses and fostering the best possible health and wellbeing.

Why Harmonizing the Chi is Important for Optimal Thymus Gland Function

Harmonizing Chi flow is crucial for the thymus gland's proper performance and, therefore, for our general health. The lymphatic system's balance and vitality are crucially maintained by Chi, the essential life force energy, with the thymus gland serving as a critical factor in the growth and control of the immune system.

Chi boosts the thymus gland's capacity to grow and generate T cells, which are essential for immunological responses when it flows easily and harmoniously. T cells can recognize and successfully attack infections and aberrant cells in the body thanks to the right education and selection provided by a healthy thymus gland. Our immune system is subsequently strengthened, improving our capacity to fend against illnesses, infections, and other health issues.

Chi flow may be balanced to support the thymus gland's healthy operation and keep it in balance. The capacity of the thymus gland to communicate with other organs and tissues in the lymphatic system is improved by a smooth and balanced Chi flow inside the gland, encouraging a harmonic interaction between the many parts of our immune system. The preservation of general health and wellbeing is made possible by this interconnectedness, which also enables effective immunological responses and appropriate immune monitoring.

Additionally, balancing Chi flow has a significant influence on our physical, mental, and emotional health. Chi may foster a state of harmony inside our body-mind system when it is balanced and flowing freely. It promotes mental clarity, eases tension, and helps regulate emotions. By guaranteeing appropriate energy distribution and assisting the body's self-healing processes, it also contributes to preserving physical health and vitality.

On the other hand, an imbalance or interruption in Chi flow may cause discord in the lymphatic system and thymus gland. Weakened immunological responses, unbalanced T cell generation, and poor general health may be caused by obstructions or shortages in Chi flow. Additionally, it may cause emotional discord, increased stress, and a loss of vitality.

The thymus gland and the whole lymphatic system may be brought back into balance and vitality by actively striving to harmonize Chi flow via techniques like Lymph-Chi Treatment. Blockages may be removed, energy channels can be revitalized, and the free flow of Chi can be encouraged by using techniques like tapping, rubbing, and applying pressure. In turn, this promotes the thymus gland's healthy operation, strengthens the immune system, and benefits our general health.

How Stress, Emotions, and Happiness Can Affect the Thymus Gland and the Repercussions of Blockages on Health

The lymphatic system as a whole as well as the thymus gland are significantly impacted by stress, emotions, and happiness. As a crucial component in the formation and control of the immune system, the thymus gland is susceptible to the effect of these factors, which may have a substantial impact on its function and, in turn, our physical, emotional, and mental health.

The thymus gland and immune system have been shown to suffer negative consequences of stress, whether it be acute or chronic. The body produces cortisol and other stress chemicals while under stress, which may inhibit immunological responses and interfere with the thymus gland's function. Stress that is prolonged or chronic may cause the thymus gland to be continuously suppressed, which impairs immunological response and reduces T cell production.

The thymus gland and the lymphatic system are influenced by emotions, both good and bad. Reduced thymus gland activity and immune system malfunction have been linked to negative emotions including fear, worry, and melancholy. On the other hand, positive feelings like pleasure, happiness, and love have been connected to better thymus gland activity and immunological responses.

Particularly, happiness has been discovered to have advantageous effects on the lymphatic and thymus systems. Happiness causes our bodies to produce neurotransmitters and chemicals that enhance general health, including immune system function. This feeling of wellbeing may increase thymus gland activity, promoting T cell development and maturation and strengthening the immunological response.

In terms of the body, obstructions in the lymphatic system may cause sluggishness, edema (swelling), and a decreased ability to remove toxins. Despite their best efforts, people may have trouble losing weight, since the lymphatic system is so important for fat metabolism and disposal. Disruptions in the lymphatic system may also lead to hormonal imbalances, which can affect the control of hormones in general as well as other aspects of reproductive health.

Blockages in the lymphatic system may cause mood swings, anger issues, increased stress, and a feeling of general imbalance on an emotional and mental level. The body-brain-mind relationship is closely related to the lymphatic system and the thymus gland in particular. This relationship may be broken by any changes in lymphatic flow, which may have an impact on mental clarity, cognitive performance, and emotional stability.

It's necessary to address these blockages and aberrations in the lymphatic pathways and Chi flow to promote holistic health and return the body's systems to their ideal state. With its methods to promote lymphatic circulation and restore Chi flow, Lymph-Chi Treatment may help clear these obstructions and balance the thymus gland. This promotes emotional stability, mental clarity, and the treatment of physical ailments, leading to an improvement in general health and vitality.

As already discussed, the thymus gland and the lymphatic system are strongly impacted by stress, emotions, and happiness. Weight problems, hormone imbalances, anxiety disorders, and cognitive impairment are just a few of the physical, emotional, and mental health effects of lymphatic system blockages and altered Chi flow. By removing these obstructions and restoring Chi flow through techniques like Lymph-Chi Treatment, we can help the thymus gland, improve general health, and restore the lymphatic system's optimal operation.

Daily Stimulation of the Thymus Gland

It is crucial to regularly stimulate and maintain the thymus gland to maximize its functionality and unlock its full potential. The reason is that it helps the lymphatic system maintain and retain vitality.

However, this section will discuss the relevance of daily thymus gland stimulation, how it may be accomplished, and the advantages it has for our physical, emotional, and mental health. We may unleash the thymus gland's full potential and advance the health, vitality, and performance of our immune systems by implementing these techniques into our everyday routines.

Restoring the thymus gland's balance and treating lymphatic system dysfunctions are both possible with Lymph-Chi Treatment. This treatment successfully restores the lymphatic system's normal operation and boosts the thymus gland's vitality thanks to its special methods and strategies.

The potential of Lymph-Chi Treatment to treat lymphatic system blockages is one of its main advantages. These obstructions, which may be brought on by physical reasons, psychological stress, or other circumstances, may obstruct lymph fluid movement and interfere with communication among lymphatic system organs, including the thymus gland. To promote lymphatic circulation, remove obstructions, and restore the normal flow of lymph throughout the body, Lymph-Chi Treatment uses methods including tapping, rubbing, and applying pressure. By doing this, it aids in removing constraints that obstruct the thymus gland's and other lymphatic organs' efficient operation.

Additionally, Lymph-Chi Treatment is essential for bringing the thymus gland back into balance. This treatment stimulates the thymus gland, improving its vitality and harmonious operation, by using specialized methods on the thymus region, such as mild pressing or circular rubbing. With the use of these focused approaches, the thymus gland is stimulated to create and mature T cells, which are crucial for a healthy immune system. Regular Lymph-Chi Treatment sessions may help the thymus gland reach its ideal condition, which will improve immunological responses and general wellbeing.

Lymph-Chi treatment offers a variety of holistic advantages in addition to treating dysfunctions and harmonizing the thymus gland. It helps the body rid itself of toxins and waste, lightening the load on the lymphatic system and improving its performance. It helps provide vital nutrients and oxygen to cells, supporting their optimum function, by enhancing lymphatic circulation.

Additionally, Lymph-Chi Treatment has a significant influence on our mental and emotional health. Emotional tension, worry, and a feeling of inner quiet and balance may all be improved when lymphatic system obstructions are cleared, and the flow of Chi is balanced. As a result of this treatment's recognition of the interdependence of the body, mind, and spirit, holistic wellbeing is supported in addition to physical health.

You may experience the transforming effects of Lymph-Chi Treatment, which include nourishing your lymphatic system, reviving the thymus gland, and increasing overall health and vitality, by including it in your wellness regimen.

Integration of Lymph-Chi Treatment with Exercises and Daily Practices to Stimulate the Thymus Gland

The efficiency of activating the thymus gland may be significantly improved by combining Lymph-Chi Treatment with physical activity and daily rituals. You may consistently support the thymus gland, encouraging its vitality and ideal functioning, by including certain methods and exercises into your daily routine.

Tapping is a crucial practice for thymus gland stimulation. You may stimulate and awaken the energy of the thymus gland by lightly pressing the region of the chest where it is situated. Start by repeatedly tapping the chest with your fingers, paying attention to the upper sternum. This tapping action promotes the thymus gland's general health by enhancing blood flow, lymphatic circulation, and Chi energy.

Rub the thymus gland in a clockwise direction as an alternative remedy. Apply light pressure and gently massage the thymus region with your fingers or the palm of your hand. This activity encourages the thymus gland's healthy activation and function. This approach may be used many times throughout the day to provide the thymus gland regular stimulation.

There are more daily routines that may help boost thymus gland stimulation in addition to these workouts. Exercises that include deep breathing, including diaphragmatic breathing, improve lymphatic circulation and oxygenate the body. You may encourage calmness, lessen tension, and support the general health of the lymphatic system, including the thymus gland, by taking slow, deep breaths.

The thymus gland may be stimulated by keeping a good outlook and practicing positive emotions like joy and thankfulness. The thymus gland and the general equilibrium of the lymphatic system may benefit by participating in enjoyable activities, practicing mindfulness, and cultivating healthy relationships. Consciously developing happy emotions may help stimulate the thymus gland, since emotions and thoughts have a significant impact on the flow of Chi in our bodies. This integrated strategy offers a holistic and all-encompassing way to encourage the thymus gland's health and the lymphatic system's general wellness.

When adopting these techniques into your everyday life, keep in mind that consistency is essential. You may benefit from these combined efforts by setting aside a little amount of time each day to assist the lymphatic system and stimulate the thymus gland. Accept the power of integration and include these self-care techniques into your routine to support the health and vitality of your thymus gland as well as your general wellbeing.

Summary:

You could apply the following helpful suggestions to daily activate the thymus gland:

1. Locate a peaceful, comfortable area where you may concentrate on stimulating your thymus gland.
2. Assume a calm, upright stance to begin. Depending on whatever is most comfortable for you, you may either sit or stand.
3. To calm yourself down and unwind your body and mind, take a few deep breaths.
4. Find the location of the thymus gland, which is in the middle of your chest, between the breastbone and the collarbone.
5. Apply light pressure over the region of the thymus gland using your fingers or the palm of your hand.
6. Start massaging the thymus gland region in a clockwise, circular manner. Depending on what seems most comfortable for you, you may either use large strokes or little, circular movements. Apply light pressure consistently.
7. Imagine that good energy and vigor are pouring into the thymus gland as you massage the region. Visualize the thymus gland being active, healthy, and performing at its peak.
8. Keep massaging the thymus gland region for another 30 to 45 seconds, or longer, if you choose. Give yourself permission to be attentive to the current moment and the feelings that are present.
9. After thymus gland stimulation, pause to recognize and appreciate the work you've done to promote your general wellbeing.

10. You may carry out this thymus gland stimulation as many times as necessary throughout the day. You may find it very helpful to include it in your morning and evening rituals.

Remember: The secret is to stimulate the thymus gland with a light touch and good purpose. It shouldn't ever hurt or be unpleasant. Pay attention to your body, then adapt the pressure and technique to your degree of comfort.

Importance of Incorporating These Daily Practices to Enhance Thymus Gland Function Alongside Lymph-Chi Treatment

To get the most out of both modalities, it's essential to combine Lymph-Chi Treatment with routines that improve thymus gland function. While Lymph-Chi Treatment offers specific methods to activate the thymus gland and regulate the lymphatic system, everyday activities operate as a constant reinforcement system, enhancing the therapeutic benefits and encouraging optimum thymus gland activity.

You may adopt a regular and proactive strategy to sustain the health of the thymus gland by participating in daily rituals like tapping, rubbing, and positive intention to stimulate the thymus gland. These techniques not only enhance the benefits of Lymph-Chi Treatment but also give you the capacity to actively participate in your own health.

The regular stimulation of the thymus gland aids in igniting its vitality, enhancing lymphatic flow, and enhancing immunological performance. The thymus gland, which is essential to general health and energy, may be kept in its ideal form with frequent attention and care.

Combining Lymph-Chi Treatment with these techniques in your daily routine encourages a synergistic result. While Lymph-Chi

Treatment sessions provide concentrated and targeted stimulation, everyday routines operate as an ongoing affirmation of the significance of the thymus gland. The lymphatic system and the thymus gland benefit from the harmonic balance that is created by this integration over the long run.

Adding regular routines also promotes a stronger sense of self-care and your relationship with your body. You may create a conscientious and proactive attitude toward your health by devoting time and attention to thymus gland stimulation. By tuning into your body's subtle changes and swiftly addressing any imbalances, you may promote general wellbeing thanks to your increased awareness.

By realizing how important a part Lymph-Chi Treatment and thymus gland function play in the growth and control of the immune system, we equip ourselves to take preventative measures to ensure optimal performance.

Lymph-Chi Treatment is recognized as a potent method for removing blockages and reestablishing the harmony of the lymphatic system and Chi flow. You can stimulate these vital organs by following the simple exercise illustrated above. These exercises will ideally promote the symbiotic interaction of the thymus gland and other lymphatic system organs, and thus ensure strong immunological responses and general vitality of the body.

Remember that our overall health and wellness are intimately connected to the lymphatic system and its components, which points to the thymus gland's efficiency, as well. Thus, we need to leverage our body's healing power to give ourselves the ability to live a healthy.

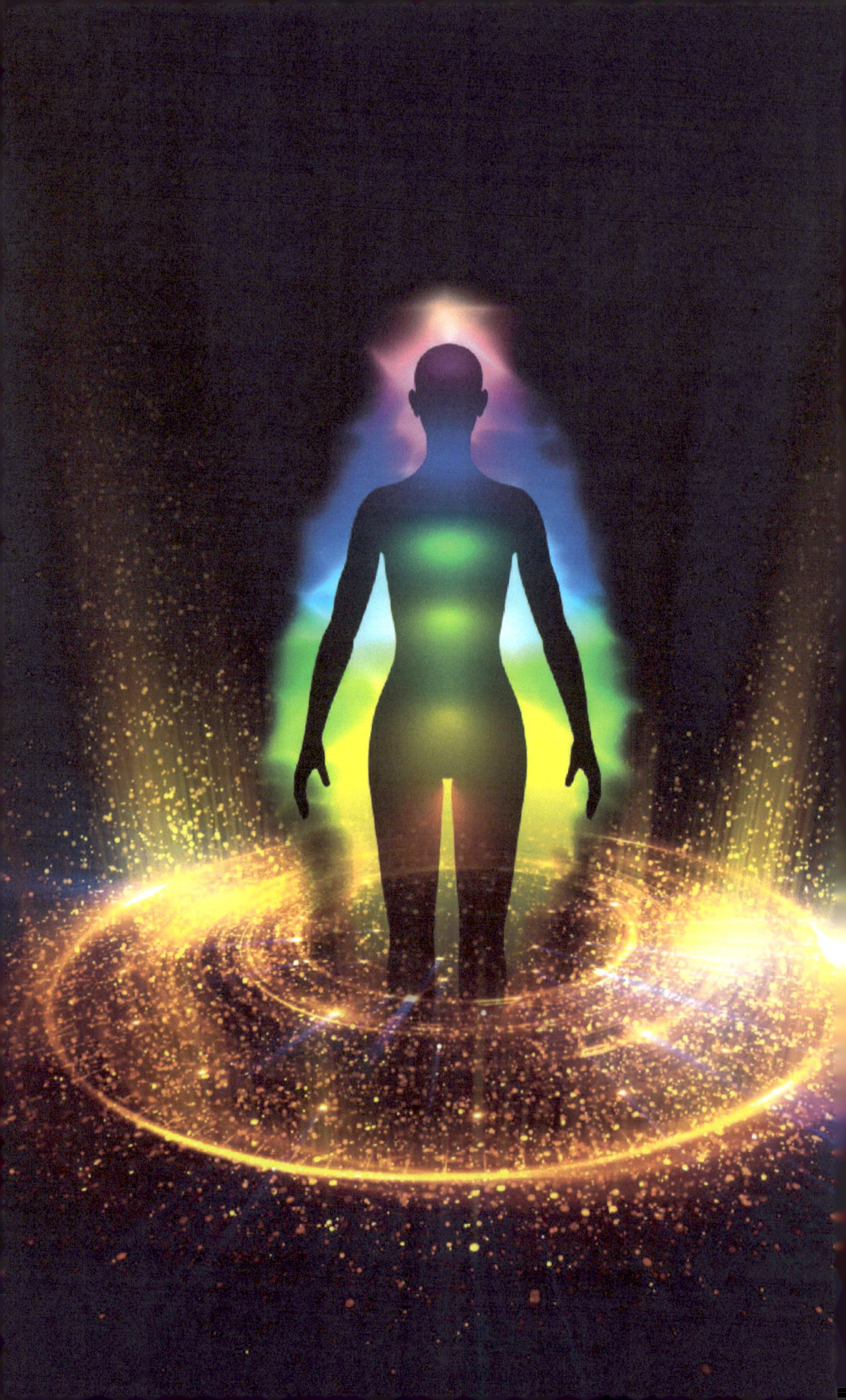

08

THE ROLE OF CHI IN PREVENTING SICKNESS

The concept of Chi is a fundamental aspect of Eastern medicine and is believed to be a vital force that flows through the body, maintaining health and vitality. When the flow of Chi is balanced, the body is healthy and free from disease. On the other hand, when Chi is blocked or imbalanced, sickness can occur. In TCM, the balance and free flow of Chi are essential for treating and preventing sickness.

The Lymph-Chi Treatment recognizes the importance of Chi in the prevention of illness and promotes the free flow of this vital energy throughout the body. By unblocking the meridians and channels that carry Chi, the Lymph-Chi Treatment helps restore balance and improve the body's natural healing abilities.

In addition to promoting the free flow of Chi, the Lymph-Chi Treatment also focuses on optimizing lymphatic function, which can help remove toxins and waste products from the body. This detoxification process is essential for preventing illness and maintaining optimal health.

By incorporating the principles of TCM into the Lymph-Chi Treatment, clients can experience a range of benefits, including improved immune system function, reduced inflammation, and a greater sense of overall wellbeing. With a focus on prevention before sickness, the Lymph-Chi Treatment offers a holistic approach to health and wellness that can help individuals maintain optimal health and prevent illness before it occurs.

In this chapter, we will explore how Chi travels through the internal organs and how blockages in these organs can lead to illness. We will also discuss the role of reading the energy system in future disease prevention and how healthcare practitioners integrate mind, emotion, body, and soul to maintain a healthy flow of Chi.

Moreover, we will delve into ways to turn up or down the energy in the body system where needed to restore balance and promote healing. So, let us dive into this fascinating topic and learn more about how to harness the power of Chi to prevent disease.

Future Prevention of Disease by Reading the Energy System

In Traditional Chinese Medicine, the focus is on maintaining the balance of Chi within the body to promote optimal health and prevent disease. One way to do this is by reading the body's Chi energy system to identify any imbalances or blockages that may lead to disease in the future.

Reading the body's Chi energy system involves using various diagnostic techniques like observation, palpation, and questions to assess the flow and quality of Chi in the body's meridian system.

Observation involves assessing the external signs of Chi imbalance, such as changes in skin color, texture, and temperature, as well as changes in facial expression, body posture, and movements. For example, a pale complexion may indicate a Chi deficiency, while a red complexion may indicate an excess of heat.

Palpation involves feeling the body for areas of tenderness, tightness, or other abnormal sensations. This can help identify areas of blockage or stagnation in the meridian system, which may lead to disease if left untreated.

Questioning involves asking the client about their symptoms, medical history, lifestyle, and emotional state. This information can help identify any underlying imbalances or stressors that may be affecting the flow of Chi in the body.

Once any imbalances or blockages are identified, the next step is to rebalance the body's Chi energy system using various Chi-based therapies, such as acupuncture, herbal medicine, Tai Chi, Qigong, and dietary and lifestyle changes.

Acupuncture involves inserting thin needles into specific points along the meridians to stimulate the flow of Chi and remove any blockages or imbalances.

Herbal medicine involves using specific herbs and formulas to nourish and strengthen the body's internal organs and balance the flow of Chi.

Tai Chi and Qigong are gentle exercises that involve slow, flowing movements, deep breathing, and meditation to improve the flow of Chi and promote overall health and wellbeing.

Food and lifestyle changes may also be recommended to support the body's Chi energy system, such as eating a balanced diet, getting regular exercise, reducing stress, and getting adequate rest and sleep.

By reading the body's Chi energy system and addressing any imbalances or blockages, it is possible to prevent any illness or hormonal dysfunction from happening in the future and promote optimal health and wellbeing.

Integrating Mind, Emotion, Body, and Soul

The principle of Lymph-Chi Treatment recognizes the importance of integrating the mind, emotion, body, and soul for overall wellness. This holistic approach acknowledges the interconnectedness of all aspects of the human experience and emphasizes the importance of addressing imbalances in each area to achieve optimal health and wellness.

Integrating the mind involves cultivating a positive and focused mental state. Negative thoughts and emotions can disrupt the flow of Chi, leading to physical and emotional imbalances. Practicing mindfulness, meditation, and visualization techniques can quiet the mind and bring it into a more centered state.

Emotional health is also crucial for overall wellness. Emotions that are not expressed or processed effectively can lead to physical symptoms and imbalances in the body's Chi energy. Practices like journaling, therapy, and energy healing can release and process emotions, thus promoting emotional balance.

The body is a physical manifestation of the mind and emotions. When we neglect our physical bodies, we create imbalances in the flow of Chi, which can lead to illness and disease. Regular exercise, healthy eating habits, and proper self-care can promote physical health and support the flow of Chi throughout the body.

Lastly, the soul is the essence of who we are. It is our connection to the universe and the source of our being. Neglecting the soul can lead to a sense of disconnection, which can manifest as physical and emotional imbalances. Practices like spiritual reflection, prayer, and energy healing can help nourish the soul and support overall wellness.

Integrating these four aspects of the human experience is essential for overall wellness and is a fundamental principle of Lymph-Chi Treatment. By addressing imbalances in each area and promoting the flow of Chi throughout the body, we can achieve optimal health and vitality.

CONCLUSION

The Lymph-Chi Treatment is a powerful and effective approach to improving physical and mental health. It has been specifically designed to address a wide range of health concerns, including chronic pain, inflammation, anxiety, depression, and even cancer-related symptoms like lymphedema.

In today's fast-paced world, it's essential to take care of our health, both physical and mental. Incorporating the Lymph-Chi Treatment into your self-care routine can help you achieve a greater sense of balance and wellbeing. The treatment is natural and non-invasive, promoting healthy circulation, energy flow, and immune function. The Lymph-Chi approach is gentle and can be customized to suit the unique needs of each individual.

The Lymph-Chi Treatment is based on the idea that the body's natural energy systems play a vital role in maintaining health and promoting healing. By working with these energy systems, the Lymph-Chi Treatment can help optimize the body's natural healing processes, leading to quicker and more effective healing for a variety of health concerns.

Rather than relying on harsh medications or invasive procedures, the Lymph-Chi treatment works with the body's natural healing mechanisms to promote health and wellbeing.

That being said, this approach to healing is highly individualized and can be customized to meet the unique needs of each client. By assessing the specific health concerns of each individual and tailoring the treatment approach accordingly, the Lymph-Chi therapist can optimize the healing process and promote long-term health and wellness.

Whether you are dealing with chronic pain, inflammation, digestive issues, or mental health concerns like anxiety and depression, the Lymph-Chi Treatment can help you achieve quick and effective healing. By promoting healthy circulation and immune function, this approach to healing can improve the overall quality of life and promote a greater sense of wellbeing.

Ultimately, by incorporating this treatment into your self-care routine, you can take an active role in promoting your own health and wellbeing. By working with your body's natural energy systems and optimizing the natural healing process, you can achieve quick and effective healing for a variety of health concerns and improve your overall quality of life.

ADVANCED PRAISES

First

Dr. Tracy is a superior healthcare professional. I came to her for lymphatic drainage and received far more in terms of my overall wellbeing. Her genuine caring, accumulated wealth of knowledge on holistic approaches to health, and her committed support have been worth more than I can express. Dr. Tracy is the kind of person who willingly spends her off hours researching additional ways to enhance the wellness of her clients. I consider myself extremely fortunate to have been referred to Dr. Tracy. At a bare minimum, I know I am healthier as a result of her expert and unique medical approach, yet she has offered so much more. Every treatment brings me closer to healing my body. She is an amazing person and is so passionate about what she does. She is the best of the best!

— Viki M. West
Santa Monica
Fashion Designer

Second

I cannot recommend Tracy enough. I initially visited her regarding a swollen lymph node under my armpit (nearly the size of a golf ball). After four sessions, it was completely drained. The bodywork was amazing, but energetically, she also healed me. I am now seeing her after my hernia surgery, after which my whole stomach was full of scarring tissue. It has been a journey of recovery while she breaks up the scar tissue by hand. Even though the healing has been painful, she gave me the hope of recovery. She has a special gift of intuitiveness and skill. It's not something I can explain; it's something you have to experience for yourself. She is the best.

— Cameron Richardson
Malibu
Mom of 3, Producer

Third

Finding Tracy has been a true blessing in my life. Her sessions have made me more aware of my body and I have seen a huge difference in how I feel. I finally feel like I am connected to and in tune with my body, recognizing when I need to rest or eat better. I can even identify what triggers the pains in my body. For example, if I am having headaches or fatigue, it is most likely related to any emotional triggers I am experiencing. A session with Tracy helps me process the emotions and pain. Sessions with Tracy have also helped me heal the sudden abdominal pains I was experiencing.

— Sandy Nunez
Huntington Park, CA
Transportation Lead

Fourth

After surgery, my doctor suggested that I get a lymphatic massage for my recovery. After a lymphatic massage from a well-known place, it just did not seem to be what the doctor ordered. I did more research online and was so fortunate to find Tracy. She is abundantly knowledgeable about post-surgical lymphatic work, and the body in general. Tracy expertly applied various modalities within her treatment that facilitated my recovery. I still see her regularly as a part of my self-care routine and I have even referred at least four or five others to her, all of whom have said, "It's been the best gift ever." One has even attempted to lure Tracy away from Los Angeles to Miami. Another close friend of mine even tried getting her to move to Brooklyn. I am forever grateful for Tracy's mind, hands, and heart. I can't imagine life without her!

— **Jennifer Baltimore**
Los Angeles, CA
Entertainment Lawyer

Fifth

Tracy is doing transformative work with her lymphatic treatment. A friend gifted me with one of her sessions and I had no idea what was in store for me. I thought I was going to experience a traditional massage. When my session was complete, I felt like a new person. Tracy has brilliantly honed her craft and exudes a warm bedside manner. She has studied, trained, and put into practice so much knowledge that compliments her skills and lymphatic treatment. My hope is that she pays it forward by training others in her methods (preferably at least one person who is Brooklyn based!), so that more people can experience the benefits of her treatment. Every time I'm headed to Los Angeles, she is one of the first appointments I confirm. She is beyond talented, an amazing healer, and an incredible human being.

— **Gabrielle Glore**
Brooklyn, NY
Creative Director

RESOURCE

To learn more about this revolutionary treatment, with details on courses and seminars, please visit our official website: www.lymphchi.com.

There, you will find updated schedules, training programs, valuable resources, and contact information. Explore the possibility of incorporating Lymph-Chi Treatments into your professional or personal wellness journey.

Join us now on a transformative healing path.

www.ingramcontent.com/pod-product-compliance
Lightning Source LLC
Chambersburg PA
CBHW040936030426
42335CB00001B/6